Antisocial Personality

'This is an exceptional book. It aims at, and achieves, a brilliant integration of population- and person-centred perspectives on this complex mental health problem. Despite the many controversies that surround the construct of ASPD, the book at all times remains balanced and highly practical, filled with deep understanding and sage advice. It is an invaluable guide through a labyrinthine field from two great masters of forensic mental health. It is simply the best book on the subject to date.'

Peter Fonagy, OBE, FMedSci, Head of Division, Psychology and Language Sciences, UCL, and Chief Executive, The Anna Freud National Centre for Children and Families, London, UK

This is a valuable book on an important topic by leading scholars with extensive front-line experience working with severely antisocial individuals. Exceptionally well written, it surpasses other available sources in its balanced and complementary coverage of conceptual-empirical and clinical-applied material. Latter chapters on treatment of antisocial behavior and psychopathy are particularly incisive and informative. The book will be of interest to researchers for its up-to-date coverage of diagnostic issues/ approaches and causal factors, and to practitioners for its nuanced consideration of prospects and obstacles in providing services to offender populations.

Christopher J. Patrick, PhD, Distinguished Research Professor of Psychology and Director of Clinical Training, Florida State University, USA

'Richard Howard and Conor Duggan are to be congratulated for this refreshing evaluation of a thorny subject. Antisocial personality disorder and its mirror twin, psychopathy, are ugly monuments despoiling the psychiatric landscape; we seem unable to do anything to make them more attractive and acceptable, and our attempts at treatment have been lamentable. But Howard and Duggan are not dissuaded. They quietly and systematically dissect the classification, neuroscience, developmental, therapeutic, and epidemiological aspects of the condition, providing valuable insights and commentary. Along the way, they illuminate aspects that we should all recognize, including the unsatisfactory and heterogeneous nature of the word "psychopathy", the strong evidence that antisociality show its colours most strongly in adolescence (when we should be intervening therapeutically), and that we have been less than bold in the evaluation of our interventions.

Those who encounter antisocial behaviour in any aspect of their work could benefit from this very readable and well-set-out book; it has messages for all of us.'

Peter Tyrer, Emeritus Professor of Community Psychiatry, Imperial College, London, and Consultant in Transformation Psychiatry, Lincolnshire Partnership NHS Foundation Trust, UK

'The authors disaggregate the antisocial personality disorder classification and present a learned and refreshing exploration of the multiple factors that are implicated in antisociality in general. Encompassing biological, psychological, social, and cultural facets, they integrate a wide literature in a fascinating and transformative appraisal. After examining treatment outcome research, they distil their knowledge, wisdom, and experience into sound practical advice for managing and treating people who can be antisocial. Academics, health and social care professionals, legal personnel, and interested members of the general public would all gain from reading this work. It is a real *tour de force*.'

Mary McMurran, Ph.D., former Professor of Personality Disorder Research,
University of Nottingham, UK

'The scholarly contributions of Dr Howard and Professor Duggan to the field of personality disorder never cease to amaze. In this book, they eloquently present an innovative framework for conceptualizing antisocial personality disorder, which is underpinned by research evidence and clinical realities. Through the prism of prosocial behaviour, this book takes our understanding of the emotional, motivational, and neurobiological determinants of human antisocial behaviour to new horizons, with some important implications for future research and clinical practice.'

Najat Khalifa, MD, FRCPsych, FRCPC, Queen's University, Canada

Antisocial Personality

Theory, Research, Treatment

Richard Howard
University of Nottingham

Conor Duggan
University of Nottingham

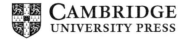

CAMBRIDGE
UNIVERSITY PRESS

University Printing House, Cambridge CB2 8BS, United Kingdom

One Liberty Plaza, 20th Floor, New York, NY 10006, USA

477 Williamstown Road, Port Melbourne, VIC 3207, Australia

314–321, 3rd Floor, Plot 3, Splendor Forum, Jasola District Centre, New Delhi – 110025, India

103 Penang Road, #05–06/07, Visioncrest Commercial, Singapore 238467

Cambridge University Press is part of the University of Cambridge.

It furthers the University's mission by disseminating knowledge in the pursuit of education, learning, and research at the highest international levels of excellence.

www.cambridge.org
Information on this title: www.cambridge.org/9781911623984
DOI: 10.1017/9781911623892

© The Royal College of Psychiatrists 2022

First published 2022

A catalogue record for this publication is available from the British Library.

ISBN 978-1-911-62398-4 Paperback

Contents

Preface

In this book, the authors – one a forensic psychologist, the other a forensic psychotherapist – attempt to understand antisocial personality, its origins and consequences. The overarching conceptual framework adopted by the authors is one that emphasises the importance of motivation and emotion for a proper understanding of antisocial personality. In short, it asks: What are the underlying emotions and motivations that drive antisocial behaviour?

The book divides into two halves. In the first half, we describe the current state of play regarding the assessment and conceptualisation of personality disorder generally, and of antisocial personality disorder (ASPD) in particular. We focus particularly on recent critiques of the nosological systems – DSM-5 and ICD-11 – that are currently used to assess personality disorder (PD). The three chapters that follow offer a distinctly psychological perspective on antisocial personality, considered first as a disorder of interpersonal function, second as a developmental disorder, and third as a neurobehavioural disorder. We attempt to answer the following questions: What is it that is lacking in 'antisocial' individuals and causes them to act in an antisocial manner? What is the characteristic interpersonal style of the antisocial individual? What are the key developmental antecedents of adult antisociality? What (if anything) can neurobehavioural studies tell us about the root causes of antisociality?

'Antisociality' generally describes behaviours that harm or lack consideration for the well-being of others. It refers to any type of conduct that violates the basic rights of another person and any behaviour that is considered to be disruptive to others in society. Antisociality can best be viewed as a spectrum that ranges from prosocial behaviour at one end of a continuum to severe antisocial behaviour at the other end. The construct of antisociality must be viewed from the perspective of the norms, values and goals that are deemed to be normative within a given cultural setting – they clearly differ from culture to culture. A fundamental premise of the authors' account is that to understand antisocial behaviour it is first necessary to understand prosocial behaviour. Why do most people, most of the time, and within a given culture, behave in a prosocial manner towards their fellow human beings and generally conform to the norms, rules and laws of society?

In the second half of the book we examine antisocial personality from a clinician's perspective. How should the clinician attempt to understand, and then treat, individuals whose behaviour has brought them into conflict with society and has led them to fall foul of the criminal justice system? In reviewing the literature – particularly regarding epidemiology and treatment – we were constrained by the fact that most of the past literature in this area has adopted a medical model and has considered antisocial personality as a disorder. As a consequence, investigations of personality pathology (one should perhaps refer to it as the outer fringes of the normal spectrum of personalities) have been overly focused on particular categories of PD on the dubious (and almost certainly false) assumption that these categories exist as real entities.

There has recently been a welcome move away from seeing PDs as categories, in favour of viewing them as collections of traits that are continuously distributed in the population. Nonetheless, the authors express the view that to understand antisocial PD it is not sufficient to enumerate a set of traits associated with 'being antisocial', albeit this might be a necessary and useful part of the assessment. Traits are purely descriptive and do not offer an adequate *explanation* of the individual's antisocial behaviour. The trick here, it is suggested, is to combine a nomothetic (trait-based) approach with an idiographic (person-centred) approach. We outline an assessment model that is based on McAdams' tripartite model of Self: as social actor, as motivated agent and as autobiographical author. 'Self as social actor' captures the personality traits that in the broader population have been found to be significantly associated with antisociality. The question here is: To what extent does this patient show these antisocial traits? The idiographic approach is captured by the last two items in the Self triad. Here the assessment will aim to capture, first, the particular motives, values and goals that drive the individual's antisocial behaviour, and second, the feeling of continuity, coherence and sense of agency expressed in the individual's life story. What were the particular incidents or turning points in this patient's life story, and how successful or unsuccessful were their attempts to deal with those incidents or turning points?

Finally, a caveat is in order. The constructs of 'antisocial personality disorder' and 'psychopathy', the topics of this book, are premised on the idea that antisocial behaviours – those that harm or lack consideration for the well-being of others – emanate from a set of personal characteristics that are in some sense aberrant or deviant (they deviate from socially and culturally accepted norms). An underlying disorder – 'psychopathic or antisocial/dissocial personality *disorder*' – may be *inferred*. Yet to describe someone as psychopathic or having an antisocial personality disorder is clearly to make a value judgement (implicitly, the person is judged to be 'difficult, unpleasant and troublesome') and this value judgement may be concealed under the guise of a diagnosis of ASPD or psychopathy. Such a value judgement does not pertain to other medical diagnoses, or even to other psychiatric diagnoses. This makes these constructs highly problematic. Necessarily, when reviewing the literature pertaining to these constructs, we have been constrained by the prevailing view that antisocial personality and psychopathy reflect some sort of underlying disorder that exists independently of the antisocial behaviours and traits with which they are associated. Such a view should not be uncritically accepted. We should be mindful of the human tendency to be all too easily seduced by verbal labels that, when habitually used to describe the world (including the people in that world), become reified in the minds of those who use them.

Chapter 1

The Nosological Background

In this book the authors explore current issues in the conceptualisation, assessment and treatment of antisocial personality. Consideration of two related constructs, psychopathy and sociopathy, is unavoidable given overlap in their meanings. The *New Oxford Dictionary of English* offers the following definition of 'antisocial': contrary to the laws and customs of society; causing annoyance and disapproval in others, e.g., aggressive and antisocial behaviour [1]. A person with antisocial personality is therefore one who both acts unlawfully or contrary to social norms and customs, and behaves in ways that others find objectionable. The dictionary defines a 'sociopath' as one with a personality disorder manifesting itself in extreme antisocial attitudes and behaviour.[1] A 'psychopath' is defined as a person suffering from chronic mental disorder with abnormal or violent social behaviour. This latter definition perhaps reflects the common (layperson's) perception of the 'psychopath' as someone who is dangerous and mentally deranged. Implicit in these definitions is the idea that there exists a continuum of antisocial behaviour or 'antisociality', ranging from the obnoxious but relatively benign, through the more severe and disordered (sociopathy) to the extreme (psychopathy) characterised by abnormal or violent social behaviour. This idea of an antisociality continuum is reflected in contemporary usage of these terms.

Lykken, a pioneer of contemporary psychopathy research, drew a distinction between the sociopathic individual or 'sociopath' and the 'psychopath' [2]. While they were said to share a lack of the restraining influence of conscience and of empathic concern for other people, Lykken contended that sociopaths' unsocialised character is due primarily to parental failures rather than inherent peculiarities of temperament; they are 'the feral products of indifferent, incompetent or over-burdened parents' [2, p. viii]. In contrast, psychopaths' inherent peculiarities of temperament make them unusually intractable to socialization. Although subsequent research has not supported Lykken's distinction between these two types of antisociality in terms of their aetiology, subsequent research reviewed by Iacono has validated the existence of aetiologically distinct variants of antisociality – primary and secondary psychopathy – that are both appreciably heritable [3]. This distinction has stood the test of time and is considered in greater detail in Chapter 4. Iacono points out that parenting, especially from fathers, is important to the socialization of children, as we will see when, in Chapter 3, we consider family factors in the development of antisocial personality.

---

[1] The term 'sociopath' was introduced by the American sociologist George Partridge in the 1930s.

All three terms – antisocial, sociopathic, psychopathic – have appeared in psychiatric nosologies, the most important of which are the various iterations of American Psychiatric Association's Diagnostic and Statistical Manual (DSM [4]) and the World Health Association's International Classification of Diseases (ICD [5]). The latter has adopted the term 'dissocial' to mean much the same as 'antisocial'. Below we will review how these various constructs have been treated in the various iterations of DSM and in ICD-11. Interesting to note at the outset is that 'psychopathy' and 'antisocial personality disorder' (ASPD) have been uneasy bedfellows, often diverging but at times merging together. Some psychiatrists (e.g., [6]) have been downright antipathetic toward the construct of 'psychopathy'. Conversely, some psychologists have been damning in their view of ASPD. Lykken, for example, stated: 'Identifying someone as "having" ASPD is about as nonspecific and scientifically unhelpful as diagnosing a sick patient as having a fever, or an infectious or neurological disorder' [2, p. 23]. Lykken considered that ASPD comprises a family of disorders, the largest and most important of which is the 'genus' of sociopaths. We return to psychopathy throughout book and will examine in greater detail the ASPD construct. We will first briefly review the historical development of the ASPD construct in the various iterations of DSM (here we draw heavily on the review by Crego and Widiger [7]).

ASPD in DSM

When the first edition of DSM (DSM-I [8]) appeared in 1952 it included a category termed 'sociopathic personality disturbance' encompassing a range of problems including sexual deviations, addictions, and a condition referred to as 'sociopathic personality disturbance: antisocial reaction' marked by persistent aggression and criminal deviance. When the first revision of DSM (DSM-II) appeared in 1968, the term 'reaction' was eliminated; sexual deviations, addictions and delinquent personality types were grouped together under 'Personality Disorders and Other Non-Psychotic Mental Disorders', which included a condition referred to as 'antisocial personality' [9]. Aligning the ASPD construct more closely with Cleckley's psychopath prototype [10], a person with antisocial personality was said to be grossly selfish, callous, irresponsible, impulsive, unable to feel guilt or to learn from experience and punishment, and to have a low tolerance of frustration. Individuals with antisocial personality were said to repeatedly come into conflict with society, to have a low frustration tolerance and a tendency to blame others for their problems. It further specified that a mere history of repeated legal or social offences was not sufficient to justify this diagnosis. The third edition of DSM [11] and its revision (DSM-III-R) saw much greater emphasis being placed on overt behaviour in its definition of ASPD. The nine items in DSM-III were childhood conduct disorder (required), along with poor work history, irresponsible parenting behaviour, unlawful behaviour, relationship infidelity or instability, aggressiveness, financial irresponsibility, no regard for the truth, and recklessness [12]. Explicit criterion sets were stipulated, with each criterion having relatively specific requirements. For example, recklessness required the presence of 'driving while intoxicated or recurrent speeding'. The intention was to obtain greater diagnostic reliability, but in doing so, validity was sacrificed. From a psychological point of view this move toward behavioural criteria was a retrograde step, since it neglected the psychological factors such as motivational and emotional goals that may underlie these behaviours. Classifying people by their actions rather than by their psychological dispositions or traits may be suitable for purposes of criminal law, but it neglects the variety of reasons for any given action [2]. Speeding can have a variety of motivations, for example, fear of missing an urgent appointment or a desire for the thrill of driving fast, and may be accompanied by quite different emotions (anxiety or exhilaration). New to the DSM-III-R criterion set was the lack of remorse, along with impulsivity or failure to plan ahead [12]. DSM-III-R shifted all of the personality disorders to polythetic criterion sets, requiring the presence of only a subset of features for an ASPD diagnosis.

The appearance of DSM-IV in 1994 marked a move away from DSM-III's and DSM-III-R's emphasis on behavioural criteria, many of which were removed [13]. It was the intention of the authors of the DSM-IV ASPD to shift the diagnosis closer to the conceptualization of psychopathy embodied in the Psychopathy Checklist (PCL) developed by Robert Hare in the early 1980s and revised (PCL-R; see Box 1.1) in 1991 [14]. This revision deleted two items from the original 22-item checklist (drug and alcohol abuse, and a prior diagnosis of psychopathy) and broadened the irresponsibility item to involve behaviours beyond simply parenting. The items of the PCL-R fall conceptually and statistically into distinguishable sets, or factors [15]. Factor 1 ('interpersonal/ affective') comprises separate interpersonal and affective facets. Factor 2 ('unstable and antisocial lifestyle') comprises lifestyle and antisocial facets. Two items shown in Box 1.1, sexual promiscuity and having many short-term marital relationships, contribute to the total PCL-R score but not to any of the factors or facets.

The criteria for ASPD in DSM-IV (and retained in the main section of DSM-5 [16]) are shown in Box 1.2. At least three criteria are required for an ASPD diagnosis. An additional requirement is evidence of childhood conduct disorder (CD), but the number

---

Box 1.1   PCL-R Items

glib and superficial charm*
grandiose sense of self-worth*
need for stimulation
pathological lying*
conning/manipulative*
lack of remorse or guilt*
shallow affect*
callous/lack of empathy*
parasitic lifestyle
poor behavioural controls
sexual promiscuity
early behaviour problems
lack of realistic long-term goals
impulsivity
irresponsibility
failure to accept responsibility for own actions*
many short-term marital relationships
juvenile delinquency
revocation of conditional release
criminal versatility

(* indicates interpersonal/affective items)

Box 1.2 DSM IV/5 ASPD Criteria

At least THREE of the following are required:

1. Failure to conform to social norms with respect to lawful behaviours as indicated by repeatedly performing acts that are grounds for arrest
2. Deception, as indicated by repeatedly lying, use of aliases, or conning others for personal profit or pleasure
3. Impulsivity or failure to plan ahead
4. Irritability and aggressiveness, as indicated by repeated physical fights or assaults
5. Reckless disregard for safety of self or others
6. Consistent irresponsibility, as indicated by repeated failure to sustain consistent work behaviour or honour financial obligations
7. Lack of remorse, as indicated by being indifferent to or rationalizing having hurt, mistreated or stolen from another

Box 1.3 DSM-IV/5 PDs

Cluster A Odd and eccentric	**Paranoid**: Distrust; suspiciousness **Schizoid**: Socially and emotionally detached **Schizotypal**: Social and interpersonal deficits; cognitive or perceptual distortions
Cluster B Dramatic, emotional and erratic	**Antisocial**: Violation of the rights of others **Borderline**: Instability of relationships, self-image and mood **Histrionic**: Excessive emotionality and attention-seeking **Narcissistic**: Grandiose; lack of empathy; need for admiration
Cluster C Anxious and fearful	**Avoidant** : Socially inhibited; feelings of inadequacy **Dependent**: Clinging; submissive **Obsessive-compulsive**: Perfectionist; inflexible

of CD criteria which had to be fulfilled was not specified. The chief difference between ASPD as defined in DSM and psychopathy as defined by PCL-R is inclusion in the latter of the interpersonal/affective features asterisked in Box 1.1. Hence ASPD is more closely related to PCL-R Factor 2 than to Factor 1. Psychopathy can be considered a more severe variant of antisociality than ASPD; thus, while about 75% of prison inmates were said to meet criteria for ASPD, only 15–25% were said to meet criteria for psychopathy [17]. These figures need to be qualified by recent results from a large database of US prison inmates [18]. Of 1,000 prison inmates, 42% met criteria for ASPD, and of 4,600 inmates, 22% met the criterion for PCL-R psychopathy (total score $\geq$ 30). Compared with offenders with ASPD only, those whose ASPD co-occurs with psychopathy show more severe criminal behaviour [19]. Those showing a triple comorbidity (ASPD comorbid with both psychopathy and borderline PD, characterized by a pervasive pattern of instability; see Box 1.3) were reported to show especially severe violence in their criminal history [20]. Thus although psychopathy appears to lie toward the high antisocial end of the prosocial-antisocial continuum, it gives rise to a more severe manifestation of antisociality when combined with ASPD and borderline PD.

By the time DSM-5 appeared in 2013, there was considerably more research concerning psychopathy than ASPD. This was due to the large impetus to psychopathy research resulting from development of the PCL-R, which, while requiring special training, did not require expertise or training in psychiatry. It again appeared to be the intention of the DSM-5 work group to shift the diagnosis of ASPD toward PCL-R and/or Cleckley psychopathy. This was explicitly evident in the proposed (but subsequently rejected) change in name from 'antisocial' to 'antisocial psychopathic'. Despite increasing indications that the features of PD are continually distributed and do not form discrete categories in nature, the APA Board of Trustees voted to retain the DSM-IV diagnostic system for personality disorders virtually unchanged in the main section of DSM-5. A brief description of each of these PDs is given in Box 1.3.

Among the many shortcomings acknowledged to attach to diagnostic categories of PD are their excessive comorbidity, their heterogeneity and their limited clinical utility. To this list may be added their impoverished and limited criteria. For example, hostility, sadism, lack of empathy, lack of insight, self-importance and power-seeking are arguably defining features of antisocial personality disorder, yet these aspects of mental life are absent from the DSM description. Contrast the truncated criteria for ASPD offered by DSM-IV/5 with the far more comprehensive description offered by Shedler and Westen [21]:

> Patients with this personality syndrome tend to take advantage of others, are 'out for number one,' and have little investment in moral values. They tend to be deceitful, to lie or mislead, and to engage in unlawful or criminal behavior. They have little empathy, appear to experience no remorse for harm or injury caused to others, and may show reckless disregard for the rights, property, or safety of others. They tend to act impulsively, without regard for consequences. They seem unconcerned with consequences and appear to feel immune or invulnerable. They tend to be unreliable and irresponsible (e.g., they may fail to meet work obligations or honor financial commitments). Patients with this syndrome try to manipulate others' emotions to get what they want. They tend to be angry or hostile, to seek power or influence over others, and to be critical of others. They appear to gain pleasure or satisfaction by being sadistic or aggressive. They may abuse alcohol. They tend to be conflicted about authority and are prone to get into power struggles. They blame others for their own failures or shortcomings and appear to believe that their problems are caused entirely by external factors. They have little psychological insight into their motives and behavior. They may have an exaggerated sense of self-importance.

Despite retaining the DSM-IV PD categories in the main section of DSM-5, it was decided to include an 'alternative DSM-5 model for personality disorders' in Section 3 of DSM-5, the section referred to as 'Emerging Measures and Models'. This alternative, hybrid model will be described below.

If ASPD is defined, at least in part, in terms of doing things that could result in arrest (criterion 1 in Box 1.2), then naturally a large number of incarcerated persons will appear to suffer from the disorder. A sharper focus on the individual symptoms listed in Box 1.2 reveals particular problems with ASPD as a diagnostic category. Thus in a study by Schnittker and colleagues, the presence and symptoms of ASPD were explored among people with varying degrees of contact with the American criminal justice system (CJS) [22]. Overall, nearly half of all respondents, who comprised 5,001 adults resident in the community, had some exposure to the CJS. Results indicated that contact with the CJS appeared to exert a disproportionate influence on an ASPD diagnosis. The prevalence of ASPD using the standard criteria (three or more of the symptoms listed in Box 1.2) was 14%. When symptom 1, failure to conform to social norms as indicated by having been arrested, was eliminated from the diagnosis, the prevalence of ASPD was reduced by more than 50%, even among formerly incarcerated persons. Some symptoms, in particular irritability/aggressiveness and irresponsibility, appeared to be linked to the presence and length of incarceration. This led the authors to suggest that the symptoms of those previously incarcerated might have been driven by their circumstance rather than by their personality. Last, and perhaps most important, criterion 7, lack of remorse, was met by only 5% of the overall sample and did not distinguish those receiving an ASPD diagnosis from those not receiving this diagnosis. Of the ASPD criteria listed in Box 1.2, only criteria 2 and 3 (deceitfulness and impulsivity) appeared to differentiate, to any substantial degree, those with from those without an ASPD diagnosis. We should note that assessment of ASPD in this study was carried out by lay interviewers rather than by mental health professionals. This might have led to the prevalence of an ASPD diagnosis in the sample being inflated. Despite its limitations, this study clearly indicates the need for a sharper focus on individual ASPD criteria so that criminality can be disaggregated from personality symptoms. Importantly, ASPD as specified in DSM does not appear to adequately capture the construct of insensitivity that, according to Tyrer [23], is one of its key features (see Box 1.4 below).

Gender Differences in ASPD

ASPD is three times more prevalent in men than in women, less than 1% of whom are reported to receive this diagnosis [24]. We should note that many gender differences have been observed in ASPD with regard to its prevalence, risk factors, aetiology, genetic underpinnings, comorbid disorders, prognosis, key traits and symptoms, and its overall presentation (summarised in Table 1 in [24]). Males and females with ASPD differ in predisposing factors, offending behaviours, deceitfulness and impulsivity (more likely in females), aggression and recklessness (more likely in males), relationship problems (more promiscuity in males, greater marital separation in females), substance misuse (common in females, but highly prevalent in males), comorbid internalising disorders (more common in females) and narcissistic PD (more common in males). These authors point out that there is still a dearth of research carried out on women with ASPD, and very little is understood about why these gender differences occur. There is a significant

---

Box 1.4   The Three I's of ASPD (after Tyrer [23])

- **Insensitivity**: the ability of some to disregard the humanity of others; to commit execrable acts against a person without any remorse. Insensitivity, lack of empathy and callousness all describe the central features of antisociality and is a prime factor in psychopathy. This insensitivity extends to insensitivity about oneself, the lack of awareness of who you are.
- **Infringement**: the violation of basic rights of others.
- **Injury**: injury and unjustified physical and mental aggression, used as a means of control.

proportion (somewhere between 30% and 50%) of female offenders with the disorder who would benefit from specific interventions and treatment programs, as well as customized assessment tools. We will consider gender differences in ASPD in greater detail when we examine its epidemiology in Chapter 5. In Chapter 3 we consider the possibility that developmental pathways to adult antisociality are gender-linked.

DSM-5 Alternative Model for Personality Disorders (AMPD)

In the Section 3 alternative model, the essential criteria to define any personality disorder are, first, moderate or greater impairment in personality functioning (criterion A) and, second, the presence of pathological personality traits (criterion B). As defined in this model, personality functioning consists of the degree to which there is an intact sense of self (involving a clear, coherent identity and effective self-directedness) and interpersonal functioning (reflecting a good capacity for empathy and for mature, mutually rewarding intimacy with others). This hybrid model requires assessment of the level of impairment in relation to six specific personality disorder types (antisocial, avoidant, borderline, narcissistic, obsessive-compulsive, and schizotypal) with the option for a diagnosis that is trait specified. Pathological personality traits are organized into five trait domains (negative affectivity, detachment, antagonism, disinhibition and psychoticism), each of which is further explicated by a set of trait facets reflecting aspects of the domain itself. A self-report instrument, the Personality Inventory for DSM-5 (PID-5), has been developed to measure these traits and their facets [25]. This trait system has been shown to correlate well with the Five-Factor Model, as shown in Figure 1.1. Watson and Clark [26] showed that the AMPD could be realigned to enhance its convergence with the Five-Factor Model of personality. A principal factor analysis based on these authors' revised PID-5 yielded a clear and well-defined 'Big Four' structure comprising neuroticism/negative affectivity, antagonism (vs agreeableness), extraversion (vs detachment) and conscientiousness (vs disinhibition). Watson and colleagues have shown that some, especially agentic, aspects of extraversion have important links to personality pathology, for example, recklessness and exhibitionism [26, 27].

The trait facets that are diagnostic for an ASPD diagnosis (criterion B) in the alternative model, together with criteria for impairment (criterion A), are shown in Box 1.5. The trait domains and facets can be measured either using the PID-5 [25] or by clinician ratings, for example, using the DSM-5 Clinicians' Personality Trait Rating Form (PTRF [28]). An interview-based instrument, the Semi-Structured Interview for Personality Functioning DSM-5 (STiP-5.1), has been developed to determine the severity of personality impairment [29]. Wygant and colleagues developed an interview-based instrument, the DSM-5 ASPD Impairment Criteria Interview, to assess impairments in identity, self-direction, empathy and intimacy in ASPD and psychopathy [30]. However, results indicated that only the measure of self-direction significantly predicted ASPD. It therefore remains to be seen whether impairments in identity/self associated with ASPD can be reliably identified and measured. We return to this question in the final section of this chapter and in the following chapter.

The AMPD includes a psychopathic features specifier for the diagnosis of ASPD associated with interpersonal/affective features of psychopathy. These features are indicated by low scores on anxiousness (from the negative affectivity domain) and withdrawal (from the detachment domain) together with a high score on attention seeking

DSMS Domain	Description	Core facets used to score the domain	Big Five/FFM counterpart
Negative affectivity	More frequent and intense experiences of negative emotions including depression, anxiety, and anger	Anxiousness; emotional lability; separation insecurity	Neuroticism
Detachment	Diminished interest and emotional responsivity to social intractions; diminished positive emotionality more generally	Anhedonia; intimacy avoidance; withdrawal	Low extraversion
Antagonism	Emotional, cognitive and behavioral styles that are self-focused rather than other-focused; involve willingness to take advantage of others and interpret others' behavior through negative and hostile lens	Deceitfulness; grandiosity; manipulativeness	Low Agreeableness
Disinhibition	Emphasis on short-term reward; difficulty delaying gratification and considering long-term implications of behavior	Distractibility; impulsivity; irresponsibility	Low conscientiousness
Psychoticism	Presence of cognitions, emotions, and behaviors that are non-normative, unusual, and idiosyncratic.	Eccentricity; perceptual dysregulation; unusual beliefs and experiences	High openness (?)

Figure 1.1 DSM-5 Section 3 domains and their Five-Factor Model counterparts. From [31].

(from antagonism). There seems little doubt that this alternative model represents a much closer alignment of ASPD with psychopathy. However, there is limited representation of PCL-R psychopathy traits in the alternative DSM-5 Section 3 model [31]. For example, grandiosity was not included within the dimensional trait description of ASPD nor even within the eventually added psychopathy specifier. Wygant and colleagues [30, 32] examined whether, in male and female offender samples, the DSM-5 alternative model of ASPD had moved closer to the traditional construct of psychopathy relative to the behaviourally oriented Section 2 model. While indicating a resounding affirmative response to this question, their results suggested that two additional trait facets, namely, grandiosity and restricted affectivity, might usefully be added to the trait facets listed in Box 1.5. Wygant and colleagues' results indicated that the psychopathy specifier facets (low anxiousness, low withdrawal and high attention seeking) aligned more clearly with interpersonal/affective features of psychopathy than did the Section 2 model of ASPD. When assessed by a self-report measure, the Minnesota Multiphasic Personality Inventory (MMPI), ASPD was associated with a broad spectrum of maladaptive personality traits and overlapped considerably with other PDs [33]. This points in the direction of a general severity dimension of PD, an aspect that is emphasised in the revised ICD assessment of PD which we consider below.

Box 1.5

BOX 1.5. Criteria for ASPD in DSM-5 Alternative Model

CRITERION A	**CRITERION B**

CRITERION A

At least moderate impairment in at least TWO of the following areas:

IDENTITY/SELF-DIRECTION

- Egocentricity
- Absence of internal prosocial standards
- Failure to conform to lawful behaviour

EMPATHY/INTIMACY

- Lack of concern for others
- Lack of remorse
- Exploitativeness
- Use of deceit
- Coercion, dominance and intimidation to fulfill interpersonal needs

CRITERION B

Elevations on at least SIX of the ASPD-specified traits from domains of:

ANTAGONISM

- Manipulativeness
- Deceitfulness
- Callousness
- Hostility

AND

DISINHIBITION

- Irresponsibility
- Impulsivity
- Risk-taking

Zimmerman and colleagues [34] highlight an important question with regard to the AMPD, namely, whether impairments in personality functioning (criterion A) and maladaptive personality traits (criterion B) provide distinct or overlapping information. Empirical findings reviewed by these authors indicated that measures of criterion A (including similar measures of personality functioning) and criterion B were highly correlated. A review by Widiger and colleagues [35] indicated considerable overlap between criterion A deficits and criterion B traits, and that criterion A may be largely redundant in the assessment of PD. However, other authors support the idea that criterion A (self/other deficits) adds importantly to the assessment of PD. Most clinicians would argue that intrapersonal and interpersonal problems are core features of personality pathology, with evidence suggesting that they co-exist and are reciprocally interrelated in PD patients [36]. It can be argued that the way self/other deficits are formulated in AMPD criterion A does not adequately capture all there is to know about the individual's sense of self and interpersonal relatedness or offer ideas on how to improve self and relational functioning. Two separate questions arise in relation to

ASPD. First, do the self and interpersonal descriptions contained in DSM-5 criterion A adequately capture the intrapsychic and interpersonal deficits shown by individuals with ASPD? Second, does a description of ASPD in terms of the trait domains and facets as captured by AMPD measures (see Box 1.5) adequately cover core features of their interpersonal deficits? In the chapter that follows we will examine in greater detail the question of what exactly are the interpersonal deficits of antisocial individuals.

ICD-11

Compared with DSM-5, ICD-11 represents a more radical departure from the categorical system of assessing PD. ICD-11 has jettisoned all PD categories in favour of assessing the level of PD severity, ranging from mild to severe, with each level of severity qualified by five trait domains (negative affectivity, disinhibition, dissociality, anankastia and detachment). One exception to ICD-11's eschewal of PD categories has been its retention of a 'borderline pattern specifier'. The definition of PD in ICD-11 is shown in Box 1.6. DSM-5 Section 3 and ICD-11 share a twofold conceptualization of severity and style, but there are noteworthy differences. First, ICD-11 does not include the possibility to assign specific PD diagnoses (except borderline PD). Second, in ICD-11 the assessment of trait domains is not a necessary part of the diagnosis; for a diagnosis of PD in AMPD, at least one maladaptive personality trait domain or facet must be in the clinically significant range. Third, the trait domain of psychoticism and its trait facets are absent from ICD-11.

Both DSM-5 AMPD and ICD-11 emphasize, in broadly similar ways, severity as an important factor in assessment of PD. While DSM-5 and ICD-11 both emphasise interpersonal dysfunction as critical to a diagnosis of PD in general, ICD-11 gives this rather more emphasis than does DSM-5. For ICD-11, the severity of interpersonal problems is a key factor in defining overall severity of PD. A classification as mildly severe requires that there should be notable problems in *many* interpersonal relationships. For a classification as moderately severe there should be marked problems in *most* interpersonal relationships. A classification as severe requires that there should be severe problems in interpersonal functioning *affecting all areas of life*.

It should be noted, however, that other features are important in defining severity of personality dysfunction in ICD-11, namely: degree and pervasiveness of disturbances in functioning of aspects of the self; pervasiveness, severity and chronicity of emotional,

---

Box 1.6 The ICD-11 Definition of Personality Disorder

- A pervasive disturbance in how an individual experiences and thinks about the self, others, and the world, manifested in maladaptive patterns of cognition, emotional experience, emotional expression, and behaviour.
- The maladaptive patterns are relatively inflexible and are associated with significant problems in psychosocial functioning that are particularly evident in interpersonal relationships.
- The disturbance is manifest across a range of personal and social situations (i.e., is not limited to specific relationships or situations).
- The disturbance is relatively stable over time and is of long duration. Most commonly, personality disorder has its first manifestations in childhood and is clearly evident in adolescence.

cognitive and behavioural manifestations of the personality dysfunction; and, most importantly, risk of harm to self or others. A questionnaire developed to measure severity according to ICD-11, the Standardized Assessment of Severity of Personality Disorder (SASPD), operationalises PD severity largely in terms of interpersonal dysfunction; for example, it includes the items 'being with others', 'trusting other people' and 'friendships' [37].

The dissociality trait domain in ICD-11 bears a close resemblance to the antagonism domain in the DSM-5 alternative model, having at its core 'disregard for social obligations and conventions and the rights and feelings of others. The traits of callousness, lack of empathy, hostility and aggression, ruthlessness, and *inability or unwillingness to maintain prosocial behaviour* are characteristically present but not always displayed at all times' [38]. As noted above, Tyrer suggested that ASPD is best characterized by the Three I's shown in Box 1.4 [23]. Tyrer and colleagues noted that 'the presence of insensitivity . . . is perhaps the strongest component of psychopathy' [38].

What Motivates Engagement with Others?

It is a characteristic of dissocial individuals, as noted in the quotation above, that they are unable or unwilling to maintain prosocial behaviour. Here we briefly consider the question of what motivates most people to maintain prosocial behaviour and to act prosocially. Clearly, whatever this is, it is lacking in people with antisocial traits. This question has been recently addressed in a series of studies carried out by Lockwood and colleagues [39, 40, 41]. Their results suggested that prosocial behaviour includes motivational and moral components, which are modulated by affective sensitivity. Their key finding was that people who showed a configuration of traits characterised by high empathy and affective reactivity were averse to harming others and were more willing to exert effort to benefit others. Lockwood and colleagues spoke of a deep *prosocial disposition* or affective sensitivity shown by people who engaged affectively with themselves and others; they were more likely to assume costs to benefit other people [40]. These authors found that high empathic concern and low emotional apathy were the strongest predictors among several affective and psychiatric traits putatively suggested to relate to prosocial behaviour; they suggested that a lack of affective sensitivity may be associated with poor social relationships seen in a high number of mental health conditions [41]. They further suggested that in order to recognize and care about others' emotions and act accordingly, people may have to be sensitive to the experience of emotions *and be motivated by them*. While most people are motivated to engage emotionally with others – presumably because such emotional engagement is, for most people, pleasant and rewarding – antisocial individuals can be presumed to lack this motivation, showing what Lockwood and colleagues referred to as 'prosocial apathy'. A similar view is expressed in a recent reformulation of psychopathy that viewed it as stemming from strategic, motivated processes [42]. This reformulation sees psychopathic individuals' lack of empathy and concern for others as reflecting a lack of motivation to care for others rather than an inability to care. The reason they are not motivated to engage empathically with others is that they do not place value on the sharing of emotions.

Recent findings from Lockwood and colleagues [43] suggest that despite declines in learning ability associated with ageing, motivation could play a role in preserving learning to help others ('prosocial learning'). These authors found an inverse relationship between psychopathy and prosocial learning, but only for older adults. This suggests that age-related differences in prosocial learning could be linked to basic shifts in individual traits and motivations over the lifespan. We will return to this issue of what motivates dissocial/psychopathic individuals at various points throughout this book.

Summary: DSM-5 and ICD-11

We can summarise the foregoing by saying that three main themes have emerged in both DSM-5 and ICD-11 with respect to how PDs are conceptualised and assessed. First, there has been an increasing focus on PD as comprising continuous rather than categorical variables. Second, there is an increasing recognition that PD varies critically along a severity dimension, from mild to severe. Third, there has been an emerging consensus that interpersonal dysfunction lies at the heart of PD. Despite these changes, there is recognition that the ways in which PD is currently conceptualised and assessed remain unsatisfactory. We turn now to examine recent critiques of DSM-5 and ICD-11, and ask the question: After ICD-11 and DSM-5, where next? In the final chapter we suggest a possible way forward.

Critiques of DSM-5 and ICD-11

Detailed critiques of the current state of play regarding the conceptualisation and assessment of PD have been offered by Clark and colleagues [44], Livesley [45] and Huprich [46]. Clark and colleagues highlighted inadequacies of the hybrid (type/trait) approach adopted in the DSM-5 alternative model. They argued that a severity diagnosis (criterion A) plus a full trait-specified description was sufficient and therefore a categorical diagnosis was superfluous. They supported this conclusion by showing that the overwhelming majority of people with pathological personalities do not fit prototypical PD-type descriptions and that their personalities are typically more complex than a categorical PD system would imply, even when they meet diagnostic criteria for a single PD. Diagnosis by PD type implies homogeneity where none, in fact, exists. This was exemplified in the case of two patients who both met categorical criteria for antisocial, borderline and narcissistic PDs but one of whom had a far broader range of maladaptive traits than the other. Attaching diagnostic labels to these patients is misleading since to do so would falsely imply that the trait constellation is the same in both cases. This recognition of what Wright and Woods have referred to as the 'staggering heterogeneity in how each individual functions' [47] has been highlighted by those who advocate a personalised (idiographic) approach to psychiatric diagnosis. This shifts the diagnostic focus to *dynamic* processes *within* individuals, with no assumption that these processes are homogeneous, even among individuals with the same diagnosis. While in its infancy, this personalised approach is likely to prove increasingly influential and is one that the current authors favour for the assessment of antisocial personality, as outlined in the final chapter.

Both Livesley [45] and Huprich [46] advocate a thoroughgoing re-evaluation of the PD construct. Both want to move the field beyond both traits and categories of PD in order to mitigate the shortcoming seen in current diagnostic systems. Both advocate a reconceptualization of PD that includes a focus on phenomenological aspects of personality pathology. Most importantly, we are urged to 'think more carefully about what personality is, and how it becomes pathological . . . It is time to evolve to the next level' [46, pp. 688–689]. Livesley too argues that a new course needs to be charted, one that, first, incorporates concepts from normal personality science and, second, includes multiple levels of explanation [45]. The latter fall into two groups: those concerned with publicly observable phenomena (neurobiology and observable behaviour) and those concerned with private mental events – cognitions, intentions, meaning systems.

Livesley [45] identifies several impediments to progress in the PD field. First, current conceptualisations of PDs – whether viewed as discrete categories or as constellations of traits – fail to do justice to the phenomenological and aetiological complexity of personality disorder.

A second impediment to progress is that current conceptualisations of PD adopt a version of the medical model and, relatedly, an essentialist philosophy – the idea that disorders have an underlying nature or pathology. For Livesley, the essentialist philosophy espoused by DSM-5 impedes a rational classification of personality disorders by encouraging 'an endless search for real types and encouraging conservative revisions by implying that when diagnostic criteria fail to function as designed, the appropriate response is to revise them rather than re-evaluate the diagnostic construct itself' [45]. Livesley's criticism was echoed by Wilshire and colleagues, who emphasised that the categorical approach to psychopathology espoused by DSM-5 rests on the dubious assumption that its symptom profiles are *meaningful indicators of the nature of* some *underlying disorder* [48]. This carries with it the further implication that we are ultimately seeking explanations phrased at the biological level of description; but Wilshire and colleagues point out that 'at least some aspects of DSM-5 disorders may be better captured at a psychological or even a social/cultural level of description' [48, p. 9]. The general thrust of the remainder of this book is that this is especially true of ASPD.

The third impediment to progress is the lack of an adequate alternative model. Livesley rejects trait-based models since traits are largely descriptive, atheoretical, and non-explanatory. Traits are not sufficient to capture individual difference dimensions adequately for clinical purposes since they focus primarily on structural and static features and neglect the personality *processes* crucial for understanding and treating PD. In short, trait models have just too many problems to provide the foundation for an official classification of PD.

A fourth and final impediment to progress is represented by extraneous (non-scientific, political) influences on the development of PD classification systems. Those tasked with revising PD classification systems were themselves heavily invested in research programmes based on the very diagnostic concepts that needed extensive revision or even outright elimination.

Livesley asserts that we need to consider what clinicians need to treat patients and what investigators need to investigate PD. Some authors regard the *clinical* goal of classification – to aid practitioners in identifying, conceptualising and treating conditions – as increasingly separate from a productive *research* classification [49]. Huprich points out that a description of a patient's traits may not be relevant to their therapy, which is designed *not* to modify trait domains or their facets but to reduce the problems that arise from internal or interpersonal distress. Moreover, a purely trait-based system may fail to offer the degree of differentiation needed to separate a personality disorder from other conditions, or indeed to differentiate qualitatively different types of personality pathology. As configured in the alternative model, ASPD shares many traits with other PDs, yet there is reason to think there may be core traits, for example, *insensitivity, lack of empathy, and callousness* (see Box 1.4), that differentiate it from other PDs. Huprich questions whether or not PD categories should be retained, and gives qualified support for their retention. He argues convincingly that the use of categorical and prototypical thinking is inevitable even within a dimensional system, for example, in the decision to classify someone with a PD as 'severe' or 'not severe' in the ICD-11 classification system. Huprich maintains that certain categories, in particular, borderline PD and ASPD, remain clinically useful and an important part of the diagnostic nomenclature.

Livesley asserts that what the clinician primarily needs to know is, first, whether a patient *has* PD and, second, *how severe* it is. He proposes a multifaceted framework that can be flexibly tailored to meet diverse clinical or research needs. Specifically, he proposes three facets. (1) The first is a diagnostic facet consisting of a definition of general personality disorder and a way to evaluate severity. Key elements are the degree of impairment to self and interpersonal functioning. (2) The second facet is a structured assessment facet consisting of clinically important personality constellations and a lexicon of specific traits and related structures and mechanisms. To capture the complexity and nuances of PD a diagnostic assessment needs to embed diagnostic features within a narrative that captures the richness of clinical presentations, including more inferential features such as *emotions, schemas, meaning systems, traits, relationships, conflicts*, and *self-problems*. (3) The third facet is a functional impairment facet consisting of four broad domains of personality dysfunction: *symptoms* (e.g., emotional intensity and reactivity, deliberate self-injury, dissociative reactions, quasi-psychotic symptoms and regressive behaviour); *regulatory and modulatory mechanisms* (emotional regulation capacity, impulse control, executive functions, metacognitive functioning and capacity for self-reflection); *interpersonal problems* (interpersonal schemas and patterns, conflicted relationships, interpersonal boundaries, and the capacity for intimacy, cooperation, empathy and altruism); and *self-pathology* (core self-schemas, experienced authenticity of self-states, stability of self-states and self-representations, and self-narrative).

A Role for Motivation in Personality Pathology

Huprich's above-mentioned challenge divides into two questions: First, what is personality? Second, how does it become pathological? In the following chapters we argue that motivation is intrinsically linked to personality – indeed, within mainstream personality psychology there is an increasing integration of motivation and personality [50]. The integration of motivational processes and motivation-related constructs into current conceptualizations of personality offers the possibility of a deeper understanding of both motivation and other components of personality (e.g., personality traits) [50]. If motivation is an intrinsic part of normal personality, it follows logically that it must also be an intrinsic part of personality pathology. Studies (e.g., [51]) have started to investigate the relationship between maladaptive personality traits, as operationalized using the DSM alternative model, and fundamental social motives. This framework assumes that different relationships are characterized by unique adaptive problems that must be managed in specific ways. Findings suggested that the individuals who scored high on the antagonism trait, which – as we shall see in the next chapter – captures a malign and distrustful interpersonal style, were motivated to seek status via dominance strategies (e.g., 'I am willing to use aggressive tactics to get my way') but were poorly motivated to protect self or others [51].

If we want to understand what people are like and why they behave the way they do, we need to look at both traits and *values* – the latter being *goals that people find desirable and use as guides for their behaviour across different situations* [52]. The use of network analysis (an alternative to factor analysis) to interrogate individual differences data has afforded new insights into how human values, together with neurobiologically derived motivations and personality traits, form a complex network structure comprising three basic dimensions of motivation: behavioural *approach* versus behavioural *inhibition*, *exploration* versus *constraint*, and *self-* or *ego-orientation* versus *social orientation* [53]. This last dimension, reflecting a combination of extraversion and agreeableness (the inverse of antagonism), clearly reflects differences between individuals in their propensity to act in an antisocial way – to contravene social norms and values.

Among the many symptoms in the Shedler–Westen Assessment Procedure (SWAP-200) rated by psychiatrists and clinical psychologists as prototypical of PD cases [54], one can discern two core interpersonal deficits: (1) a readiness to interact with others *but in maladaptive, self-defeating or antisocial ways* and (2) a disengagement from interaction with others, motivated by *fear of the consequences of social engagement* (see Figure 1.2). The PDs listed on the left side of Figure 1.2 all show a disposition to *engage* interpersonally, but in self-defeating and antisocial ways, while the PDs listed on the right are disposed to *disengage* interpersonally in maladaptive ways. This schema essentially re-describes PD in terms of an 'approach versus withdrawal' dimension that is fundamental to human motivation, and specifies particular motivations driving 'approach' and 'withdrawal', that is, specific fears and specific approach-based motives. It has the advantage that it knits together into a single schema the two aspects of impaired interpersonal functioning, namely, impaired capacity for intimacy and impaired socialization, and relates these to particular categories of PD.

Recalling how PDs are arranged in the three clusters shown in Box 1.3, it will be noted that Cluster B PDs align in the left-hand column of Figure 1.2, while Cluster A and C PDs align in the right-hand column. Some PDs (borderline, histrionic, narcissistic) appear in both columns, indicating that they can be associated, at different times, with both maladaptive engagement and maladaptive disengagement. Narcissism, for example, bifurcates into two related but distinct dimensions, narcissistic grandiosity (marked by boldness and *approach*) and vulnerability (marked by reactivity and *aversion*) [55].

It is apparent from inspection of Figure 1.2 that the PDs listed in the left-hand column are, broadly speaking, externalizing disorders, while the PDs listed in the right-hand column are internalizing disorders. It was recently suggested that externalizing pathology might involve inappropriate *wanting* – and acquisition – of rewards (vs sharing resources fairly), whereas internalizing psychopathology might involve insufficient *enjoyment* of experiences that most people find pleasurable [56]. Thus what all the PDs shown in the left-hand column of Figure 1.2 might have in common is their inappropriate and antisocial *desires*, for example, a desire to gratify oneself at another's expense (ASPD), or to dominate another (narcissistic PD). We speculate that this may be driven by an over-active but dysfunctional approach motivational system and an over-active dominance motivation system [57].

Motive for interpersonal engagement	PD	Motive for interpersonal disengagement	PD
Seeks pleasure from being sadistic/aggressive/ exploitative towards others	Antisocial	Fears being taken advantage of, betrayed or victimised	Paranoid Schizoid
Seeks quick/intense relationships; seeks attention of others, sometimes in a flirtatious manner	Histrionic Dependent	Fears being embarrassed or humiliated in social situations	Schizoid Schizotypal Paranoid Avoidant
Seeks power and influence over others in a controlling & competitive way. Engages in exploitative and self-serving relationships focused on personal pleasure	Grandiose Narcissism	Fears situations where might be marginalised	Paranoid Schizoid
Seeks reassurance and approval from others to an excessive degree	Borderline Dependent	Fears being rejected, excluded or abandoned	Borderline Histrionic Avoidant Dependent
Seeks confrontation – gets into power struggles	Histrionic Borderline Antisocial Narcissistic	Fears social criticism and loss of self-worth	Vulnerable narcissism

Figure 1.2 Motives for interpersonal engagement versus disengagement associated with different personality disorders. Interpersonal symptoms of PD from SWAP-200 were identified by the current authors from those deemed prototypical of actual PD cases by a national sample of psychiatrists and clinical psychologists (54).

It is perhaps unsurprising that borderline PD appears in both columns of Figure 1.2, since it combines elements of both externalizing and internalizing [58]. As a complex form of personality pathology, borderline PD putatively combines pathological desires with a pathological inability to derive pleasure (anhedonia). Several lines of evidence are consistent with the idea that anhedonia underlies the maladaptive disengagement shown by all the PDs shown in the right-hand column of Figure 1.2. First, anhedonia is an important and often overlooked symptom of borderline PD that contributes significantly to its severity [59]. Second, individuals with predominantly borderline features apparently lack the motivation to engage with their environment, including their social environment. For example, when experiencing a lack of positive affect (when feeling anhedonic) they experience a lack of 'willpower' [60]. Third, the relationship between depression and aggressive and antisocial acts (lying, stealing and violating the rights of others) is explained by individual differences in anhedonia, putatively associated with weaker inhibitory control over aggressive and antisocial impulses [61].

How Does Personality Become Pathological?

An answer to the second question raised by Huprich – how does personality become pathological? – requires a lifespan developmental approach to personality pathology and – in the current context – to antisocial personality. Other than perhaps in their early/mid-adolescent years, most people behave more or less prosocially. They are prepared, at least to a degree, to sacrifice their own self-interest in the service of acting in such a way as to benefit others. This is commensurate with *Homo sapiens* being an essentially prosocial (or 'ultrasocial') species whose mental apparatus evolved in our remote ancestors as an adaptation to the pressures of living in social groups. An evolutionary perspective suggests that the human brain is essentially a motivational device that has been shaped by evolutionary processes to promote adaptive behavioural responses to the sorts of recurring opportunities and challenges that humans have faced throughout the course of evolutionary history [50]. Yet some individuals, a minority, emerge from their teenage years as antisocial – they show a lifelong disregard for social norms and conventions, often break the law, show an aggressive and intrusive interpersonal style and sometimes show violence toward others. They often show the hallmark features of ASPD – the Three I's shown in Box 1.5. We need to know what goes wrong, when and how; and our 'how' explanation needs to include the different levels of explanation referred to above, none of which, as Livesley points out, is more important or fundamental than the rest.

Finally, problems of 'selfhood', as we have seen above, are regarded as an intrinsic part of personality pathology and are thought, in some way, to be linked to the interpersonal problems that are so characteristic of people who are classed as personality disordered. Regarding self/other functioning, Huprich suggests that the way self/other functioning is represented in DSM-5 and ICD-11 'may not adequately capture all there is to know about the individual's sense of self and interpersonal relatedness or offer ideas on how to improve self and relational functioning' [46]. Current conceptualisations of PD lack a well-worked-out theory of self, and an explanation of how self-dysfunction (however defined) is related to interpersonal dysfunction. A coherent, psychologically informed theory about what constitutes 'self' has until recently not been available. The self is first and foremost an inherent duality of I and Me, as was acknowledged years ago by the American psychologist William James. We will argue with McAdams [62] that psychologically speaking, the I/Me dynamic plays out in three different guises: the self as (1) social actor, (2) motivated agent and (3) autobiographical author. Stated succinctly, to know the self fully is to know the traits, the goals and the stories. We will therefore attempt to examine the question of what aspect(s) of self might be abnormal in relation to antisocial personality. This will necessarily be speculative since there is a lack of empirical data addressing this aspect of functioning in people with ASPD.

The chapters that follow are premised on the idea that PDs, like all mental disorders, are complex, multi-factorial problems which can be understood and approached from a variety of perspectives. We offer three complementary perspectives of antisocial personality: an interpersonal perspective, a developmental perspective and a neurobehavioural perspective. We then consider antisocial personality in clinical contexts, particularly in regard to its treatment, and examine ethical and legal issues arising from the treatment of people with ASPD. As will become clear as we proceed, we regard antisociality as being a continuum of severity, running from an 'extremely prosocial' pole at one end to an 'extremely antisocial' pole at the opposite end. Not only do individuals differ in regard to their position on this continuum; they may also move along it in the course of their lives. For example, most people move toward the antisocial pole as they enter adolescence but soon return to a prosocial position. At the extreme antisocial end of the continuum are to be found individuals whose antisociality is both serious and persistent throughout the lifespan, often involving interpersonal violence.

References

1. *The New Oxford Dictionary of English.* Oxford: Clarendon Press, 1998.

2. D. T. Lykken. *The Antisocial Personalities.* Hillsdale, NJ: Lawrence Erlbaum, 1995.

3. W. G. Iacono. A Minnesota perspective on Lykken's 'Psychopathy, sociopathy, and antisocial personality disorder'. In: C. J. Patrick, ed., *Handbook of Psychopathy*, 2nd ed. New York: Guilford Press, 2018; 33–38.

4. American Psychiatric Association. *Diagnostic and Statistical Manual of Mental Disorders*, 5th ed. Arlington, VA: American Psychiatric Association, 2013.

5. World Health Organization. (2018). *International Classification of Diseases for Mortality and Morbidity Statistics (11th Revision)*, 2018. www.who.int/classifications/icd/en/ (accessed 19 June 2020).

6. P. E. Mullen. On building arguments on shifting sands. *Philosophy, Psychiatry, & Psychology* 2007; **14**: 143–147.

7. C. Crego, T. A. Widiger. Psychopathy and the DSM. *Journal of Personality* 2014. https://doi.org/10.1111/jopy.12115.

8. American Psychiatric Association. *Diagnostic and Statistical Manual of Mental Disorders*. Washington, DC: American Psychiatric Publishing, 1952.

9. American Psychiatric Association. *Diagnostic and Statistical Manual of Mental Disorders*, 2nd ed. Washington, DC: American Psychiatric Publishing, 1968.

10. H. Cleckley. *The Mask of Sanity.* Oxford: Mosby, 1974/1976.

11. American Psychiatric Association. *Diagnostic and Statistical Manual of Mental Disorders*, 3rd ed. Washington, DC: American Psychiatric Publishing, 1980.

12. American Psychiatric Association. *Diagnostic and Statistical Manual of Mental Disorders*, 3rd ed., rev. Washington, DC: American Psychiatric Publishing, 1987.

13. American Psychiatric Association. *Diagnostic and Statistical Manual of Mental Disorders*, 4th ed. Washington, DC: American Psychiatric Publishing, 1994.

14. R. D. Hare. *The Hare Psychopathy Checklist – Revised*, 2nd ed. North Tonawanda, NY: Multi-Health Systems, 2003.

15. R. D. Hare, C. S. Neumann, A. Mokros. The PCL-R assessment of psychopathy: Development, properties, debates, and new directions. In: C. J. Patrick, ed., *Handbook of Psychopathy*. New York: Guilford Press, 2018; 39–79.

16. American Psychiatric Association. *Diagnostic and Statistical Manual of Mental Disorders*, 5th ed. Washington, DC: American Psychiatric Publishing, 2013.

17. R. D. Hare. Psychopathy: A clinical construct whose time has come. *Criminal Justice and Behavior* 1996; **23**: 25–54.

18. Monika Dargis, personal communication, 14 July 2020.

19. R. E. Riser, D. S. Kosson. Criminal behavior and cognitive processing in male offenders with antisocial personality disorder with and without comorbid psychopathy. *Personality Disorders: Theory, Research, and Treatment* 2013; **4**: 332–340.

20. R. C. Howard, N. Khalifa, C. Duggan. Antisocial personality disorder comorbid with borderline pathology and psychopathy is associated with severe violence in a forensic sample. *The Journal of Forensic Psychiatry & Psychology* 2014; **25**: 658–672.

21. J. Shedler, J. D. Westen. Refining personality disorder diagnosis: Integrating science and practice. *American Journal of Psychiatry* 2004; **161**: 1350–1365.

22. J. Schnittker, S. H. Larimore, H. Lee. Neither mad nor bad? The classification of antisocial personality disorder among formerly incarcerated adults. *Social Science & Medicine* 2020; **264**: 113288.

23. P. Tyrer, A. Farnam, A. Zahmatkesh, R. Sanatinia. Conceptual and definitional issues. In: D. W. Black, N. Kolla, eds., *Textbook of Antisocial Personality Disorder*. Washington, DC: American Psychiatric Press, 2021.

24. B. Bishop, B. Völlm, N. Khalifa. Women with antisocial personality disorder. In: D. W. Black, N. Kolla, eds., *Textbook of Antisocial Personality Disorder*. Washington, DC: American Psychiatric Press, 2021.

25. R. F. Krueger, N. R. Eaton, L. A. Clark, et al. Deriving an empirical structure of personality pathology for DSM-5. *Journal of Personality Disorders* 2011; **25**: 170–191.

26. D. Watson, L. A. Clark. Personality traits as an organizing framework for personality pathology. *Personality and Mental Health* 2019; **14**: 51–75.

27. D. Watson, S. Ellickson-Larew, K. Stanton, et al. Aspects of extraversion and their associations with psychopathology. *Journal of Abnormal Psychology* 2019; **128**: 777–794. https://doi.org/10.1037/abn0000459.

28. American Psychiatric Association. *Changes to the Reformulation of Personality Disorders for DSM-5*. Washington, DC: American Psychiatric Association, 2011.

29. J. Hutsebaut, J. H. Kamphuis, D. J. Feenstra, L. Weekers, H. de Saeger. Assessing DSM-5–oriented level of personality functioning: Development and psychometric evaluation of the Semi-Structured Interview for Personality Functioning DSM-5 (STiP-5.1). *Personality Disorders: Theory, Research and Treatment* 2016: **7**: 192–197.

30. D. B. Wygant, M. Sellbom, C. E. Sleep, T. D. Wall, K. C. Applegate, R. F. Krueger, C. J. Patrick. Examining the DSM-5 alternative personality disorder model operationalization of antisocial personality disorder and psychopathy in a male correctional sample. *Personality Disorders: Theory, Research, and Treatment* 2016; **7**: 229–239. https://doi.org/10.1037/per0000179.

31. J. D. Miller, C. Sleep, D. R. Lynam. DSM-5 alternative model of personality disorder: Testing the trait perspective captured in criterion B. *Current Opinion in Psychology* 2018; **21**: 50–54.

32. D. B. Wygant, J. E. Engle, M. Sellbom. Further examination of DSM-5 antisocial personality disorder and psychopathy: Findings from a female correctional sample. *Personality & Mental Health* 2020; **14**: 388–398.

33. M. Sellbom, T. A. Brown, R. M. Bagby. Validation of MMPI-2–RF personality disorder spectra scales in a psychiatric sample. *Psychological Assessment* 2020; **32**, 3: 314–320.

34. J. Zimmermann, A. Kerber, K. Rek, C. J. Hopwood, R. F. Krueger. A brief but comprehensive review of research on the alternative DSM-5 model for personality disorders. *Current Psychiatry Reports* 2019; **21**: 92.

35. T. Widiger, B. Bach, M. Chmielewski, L. A. Clark, C. DeYoung. Criterion A of the AMPD in HiTOP. *Journal of Personality Assessment* 2019; **101**: 345–355.

36. J. E. Beeney, S. A. Lazarus, M. N. Hallquist, S. D. Stepp, A. G. C. Wright, L. N. Scott, R. A. Giertych, P. A. Pilkonis. Detecting the presence of a personality disorder using interpersonal and self-dysfunction. *Journal of Personality Disorders* 2018; **32**: 1–20.

37. B. Bach, J. L. Anderson. Patient-reported ICD-11 personality disorder severity and DSM-5 level of personality functioning. *Journal of Personality Disorders*. e-View ahead of print. 2018. https://doi.org/10.1521/pedi_2018_32_393.

38. P. Tyrer, G. M. Reed, M. Crawford. Classification, assessment, prevalence, and effect of personality disorder. *Lancet* 2015; **385**: 717–726.

39. P. L. Lockwood, M. Hamonet, S. H. Zhang, A. Ratnavel, F. U. Salmony, M. Husain, M. A. J. Apps. Prosocial apathy for helping others when effort is required. *Nature Human Behaviour* 2017; **1**: 0131.

40. P. L. Lockwood, Y.-S. Ang, M. Husain, M. J. Crockett. Individual differences in empathy are associated with apathy motivation. *Scientific Reports* 2017; **7**: 17293.

41. L. S. Contreras-Huerta, P. L. Lockwood, G. Bird, M. A. J. Apps, M. J. Crockett. Prosocial behavior is associated with transdiagnostic markers of affective sensitivity in multiple domains. *Emotion*. Advance online publication. http://dx.doi.org/10.1037/emo0000813.

42. L. L. Groat, M. S. Shane. A motivational framework for psychopathy. Toward a reconceptualization of the disorder. *European Psychologist* 2020; **25**: 92–103. https://doi.org/10.1027/1016-9040/a000394.

43. J. Cutler, M. Wittmann, A. Abdurahman, L. Hargitai, D. Drew, M. Husain, P. Lockwood. Ageing disrupts reinforcement learning whilst learning to help others is preserved. *bioRxiv* 2020.12.02.407718. https://doi.org/10.1101/2020.12.02.407718.

44. L. A. Clark, E. N. Vanderbleek, J. L. Shapiro, H. Nuzum, X. Allen, E. Daly, et al. The brave new world of personality disorder-trait specified: Effects of additional definitions on coverage, prevalence, and comorbidity. *Psychopathology Review* 2015; **2**: 52–82.

45. W. J. Livesley. Why is an evidence-based classification of personality disorder so elusive? *Personality & Mental Health* 2021; **15**: 8–25.

46. S. K. Huprich. Moving beyond categories and dimensions in personality pathology assessment and diagnosis. *The British Journal of Psychiatry* 2018; **213**: 685–689. doi: 10.1192/bjp.2018.149.

47. A. G. C. Wright, W. C. Woods. Personalized models of psychopathology. *Annual Review of Clinical Psychology* 2020; **16**: 49–74.

48. C. E. Wilshire, T. Ward, S. Clack. Symptom descriptions in psychopathology: How well are they working for us? *Clinical Psychological Science* 2021; **9**: 323–339.

49. R. K. Blashfield, J. W. Keeley, E. H. Flanagan, S. R. Miles. The cycle of classification: DSM-I through DSM-5. *Annual Review of Clinical Psychology* 2014; **10**: 25–51.

50. V. Zeigler-Hill, J. K. Vrabel, D. Sauls, M. J. Lehtman. Integrating motivation into current conceptualizations of personality. *Personality and Individual Differences* 2019; **147**: 1–7.

51. V. Zeigler-Hill, K. A. Hobbs. The darker aspects of motivation: Pathological personality traits and the fundamental social motives. *Journal of Social and Clinical Psychology* 2017; **36**: 87–107.

52. R. Fischer. *Personality, Values, Culture: An Evolutionary Perspective*. Cambridge: Cambridge University Press, 2017.

53. R. Fischer, J. A. Karl. The network architecture of individual differences: Personality, reward sensitivity and values. *Personality and Individual Differences* 2020; **160**: 109922.

54. J. Shedler, D. Westen. The Shedler–Westen Assessment Procedure (SWAP): Making personality diagnosis clinically meaningful. *Journal of Personality Assessment* 2007; **89**: 41–55.

55. Z. Krizan, A. D. Herlache. The narcissism spectrum model: A synthetic view of narcissistic personality. *Personality and Social Psychology Review* 2018; **22**: 3–31.

56. D. Watson, L. A. Clark. Personality traits as an organizing framework for personality pathology. *Personality and Mental Health* 2019; **14**: 51–75.

57. S. L. Johnson, L. J. Leedom, L. Muhtadie. The dominance behavioral system and psychopathology: Evidence from self-report, observational, and biological studies. *Psychological Bulletin* 2012; **138**: 692–743.

58. N. R. Eaton, R. F. Krueger, K. M. Keyes, A. E. Skodol, K. E. Markon, B. F. Grant, D. S. Hasin. Borderline personality disorder comorbidity: Relationship to the internalizing-externalizing structure of common mental disorders. *Psychological Medicine* 2011; **41**: 1041–1050.

59. M. A. E. Marissen, N. Arnold, I. H. A. Franken. Anhedonia in borderline personality disorder and its relation to symptoms of impulsivity. *Psychopathology* 2012; **45**: 179–184. doi: 10.1159/000330893.

60. A. M. Heiland, J. C. Veilleux. Severity of personality dysfunction predicts affect and self-efficacy in daily life. *Personality Disorders: Theory, Research, and Treatment* 2021. https://doi.org/10.1037/per0000470.

61. T. Salem, E. S. Winer, D. G. Jordan, M. R. Nadorff. Anhedonia and the relationship between other depressive symptoms and aggressive behavior. *Journal of Interpersonal Violence* 2018. doi: 10.1177/0886260518770646.

62. D. P. McAdams. Psychopathology and the self: Human actors, agents, and authors. *Journal of Personality* 2020; **88**: 146–155.

Interpersonal Perspective

Chapter 2

We saw in the previous chapter that a consensus is forming around the idea that interpersonal problems lie at the heart of PD. Among researchers who have suggested that personality disorders are fundamentally disorders of relating with others are Rutter [1], Benjamin [2], Hopwood and colleagues [3] and Kiesler [4]. Conceptualizing personality pathology as fundamentally reflecting disturbances in how individuals view themselves in relation to others, and the quality of their interpersonal interactions, provides a theoretically and clinically meaningful way to differentiate personality pathology from other forms of psychopathology.

In this chapter we examine in greater detail what is known about the interpersonal style of people with antisocial personality. In the previous chapter we noted that most people are motivated to engage emotionally with others, presumably because such emotional engagement is, for most people, pleasant and rewarding. In this chapter we examine more closely the nature of the 'prosocial apathy' shown by antisocial individuals who, it might be presumed, lack the normal motivation for engaging with others. However, their goals when interacting with others may simply be different from those of most people; in which case, what are they?

Psychopathy

We also saw in the previous chapter how, particularly in the DSM-5 alternative model, the ASPD construct has been broadened to include features of psychopathy. We start by briefly reviewing the current state of play regarding the psychopathy construct, which as we saw in the previous chapter, has relied for its operationalisation on the PCL-R, the so-called gold standard measure of psychopathy [5]. While the PCL-R has been important in stimulating a wealth of research on psychopathy over the past 30–40 years, its shortcomings have become increasingly apparent. First, as a global construct psychopathy has been shown to be very heterogeneous. In a recent review, the authors stated: 'The extant literature is clear that psychopathy is multidimensional rather than taxonic, and the term "psychopath" almost certainly does not denote a homogeneous group of individuals' [6]. PCL psychopathy masks the existence of numerous subtypes among criminal samples when its individual facets are considered (e.g., [7, 8]). Only one of these subtypes, labelled *psychopathic traits offenders* by Driessen and colleagues and *prototypic psychopathy* by Krstic and colleagues, scores high across all PCL-R facets. In a study of prison inmates, some high PCL-R scorers were distinguished by high positive affect, others by high negative affect, and these two groups showed a different constellation of criminal and other correlates [9].

The second shortcoming of the PCL-R is that it comprises an unhelpful conglomeration of traits (e.g., grandiosity, selfishness) and behaviours (e.g., antisocial, irresponsible and parasitic lifestyle), thereby confounding the behaviours that we might wish to explain (crime and violence) with the variables (traits) that might explain such behaviours. Last, development and validation of the PCL in criminal samples resulted in its items being biased in favour of disinhibitory psychopathology, and in conceptual drift away from the Cleckleyan 'psychopath' prototype [10, 11]. We will also examine how antisociality relates to a broader and more recently introduced construct labelled the 'dark tetrad', comprising – in addition to psychopathy – Machiavellianism, narcissism and sadism. We will focus particularly on sexual sadism, which bears a close relationship with psychopathy [12]. Narcissism, too, is closely linked to psychopathy both conceptually and empirically [11].

Narcissism/grandiosity is, we argue, a core personality facet of psychopathy, which together with callousness/meanness and impulsiveness/disinhibition, form a 'psychopathy triad'. This triadic conceptualisation of psychopathy is consistent both with the Triarchic Psychopathy Model (TPM) introduced by Patrick and colleagues [13] and with Salekin's [14] review of child psychopathy that emphasized its three dimensions: grandiose-manipulative, callous-unemotional and daring-impulsive. The TPM comprises three phenotypic components: meanness (deficient empathy, lack of affiliative capacity and contempt toward others), boldness (social dominance, low stress reactivity, thrill and adventure seeking) and disinhibition (impulsivity combined with negative emotionality or 'emotional impulsiveness'). These three components of TPM, operationalised using the Triarchic Psychopathy Measure (TriPM) scales, are thought to relate in different ways to the two PCL-R factors [15]. Factor 1 (interpersonal/affective) combines meanness along with some aspects of boldness, whereas Factor 2 (unstable and antisocial lifestyle) combines disinhibition with some aspects of meanness. Thus meanness is common to both Factors 1 and 2 and accounts for their overlap. Variance in boldness and meanness unique to Factor 1 accounts for its differential relation to other disorders, for example, its association with narcissistic and histrionic personality disorders. Disinhibition correlates quite highly with meanness ($r = 0.34$–0.69) and is chiefly distinguishable from it by virtue of correlating highly and positively with all facets of neuroticism and negatively with facets of conscientiousness [16]. In a Portuguese community sample, Paiva and colleagues found that both disinhibition and meanness were positively associated with anger/hostility, physical and verbal aggression, low empathy and low agreeableness [17].

Of the three components of TPM, disinhibition appears to be most clearly linked with general psychopathology. Gottfried and colleagues found that disinhibition was associated with a history of abuse in childhood, suicidal behaviour, internalizing dysfunction, problems associated with alcohol and drug use, family history of mental illness, prison disciplinary reports for violence, number of previous criminal charges, and anger [18]. Similarly, in a large sample of juveniles undergoing court-ordered evaluations, disinhibition was associated with a range of externalizing, internalizing and social maladjustment variables [19]. Importantly, among the TriPM scales, disinhibition was reported to discriminate most efficiently between a clinically mixed forensic psychiatric sample (21% had ASPD) and a community sample [20].

Some have argued that boldness is not properly construed as a feature of psychopathy, since it has been found to be associated with healthy adjustment and prosocial functioning. There can be no doubt, however, that boldness was a feature of Cleckley's prototypical psychopath. Patrick has convincingly argued that the masked pathology that Cleckley described reflects the co-occurrence of boldness and disinhibition [21]. Underscoring its association with grandiosity, boldness was associated with an inflated self-presentation in German prison inmates undergoing a PCL-R interview [22]. This means that they presented themselves as special, unique or superior to others [23]. Supporting the idea that boldness is essential to the psychopathy construct, recent evidence showed that when conjoined with even mild to moderate levels of meanness and disinhibition, boldness can manifest in callousness, domineering behaviour and a very high inclination to break the law or violate the rights of others [19]. South has, importantly, pointed out that in the context of meanness and disinhibition, boldness has *functionality*: 'boldness does not become maladaptive, rather the antagonistic and disinhibited person can *use* boldness to accomplish his or her aims' [24, p. 638].

It seems reasonable to conclude that when combined with a motivational orientation that, in Chapter 1, was referred to as *self- or ego-oriented*, boldness will manifest in a personality style that includes manipulative and potentially hostile features. Individuals with these features would be at an advantage when it comes to achieving goals of self-gratification and dominance at the expense of others, if only because they will likely persist in the face of initial rejection.

Interpersonal Style and Antisocial Personality

Interpersonal style is defined by one's characteristic approach to interpersonal situations and relationships. It includes attitudes toward, behaviours in and goals for relationships; cognitions about the meaning of relationships; affect and behaviour in interpersonal interactions; and interpretation of others' interaction behaviours [25].

Along with other factors, one's characteristic interpersonal style determines the quality of functioning in specific relationship domains, including with one's children, parents, siblings, peers and romantic partners. Interpersonal style is typically measured using the interpersonal circumplex model of interpersonal behaviour, defined by orthogonal dimensions *affiliation* (hostility vs warmth) and *dominance* (domineering vs nonassertive). The circumplex model of interpersonal style is a useful means of conceptualizing, organizing and assessing individuals' and groups' characteristic approach toward interpersonal interactions. Descriptions of maladaptive interpersonal traits in the interpersonal circumplex are shown in Box 2.1 (from [25]).

Interpersonal Style within a Hierarchical Structure of Personality Pathology

In assessing PD using the International Personality Disorder Examination (IPDE) in mentally disordered offenders, Blackburn and colleagues identified two higher-order personality dimensions, 'acting out' and 'anxious-inhibited' [26]. These dimensions, shown in Figure 2.1, together accounted for most PDs. 'Acting out' is primarily characterised by externalizing features of PD and includes symptoms of antisocial, narcissistic and histrionic PDs together with externalizing features of borderline PD (impulsivity, inappropriate anger) and features of childhood conduct disorder. It therefore corresponds closely to those PDs shown on the left-hand side of Figure 1.2 in Chapter 1 as putatively associated with *maladaptive interpersonal engagement*. 'Anxious-inhibited' is

Box 2.1 Interpersonal Style Description

Domineering: Tendency to control, manipulate, be aggressive toward, or try to change others

Vindictive: Tendency toward distrust and suspicion of others; an inability to care about the needs and happiness of others

Cold: Tendency to have difficulty expressing affection toward or feeling love for others; an inability to be generous to, get along with or forgive others

Socially avoidant: Tendency to feel anxious and embarrassed with others; difficulty expressing feelings and socializing with others

Non-assertive: Tendency to have difficulty expressing needs, acting authoritatively, or being firm and assertive with others

Exploitable: Tendency to have difficulty feeling and expressing anger to others; gullible and easily taken advantage of by others

Overly nurturant: Tendency to try to please others; overly generous to, trusting of, caring toward and permissive of others

Intrusive: Tendency toward inappropriate self-disclosure and attention-seeking; difficulty being alone

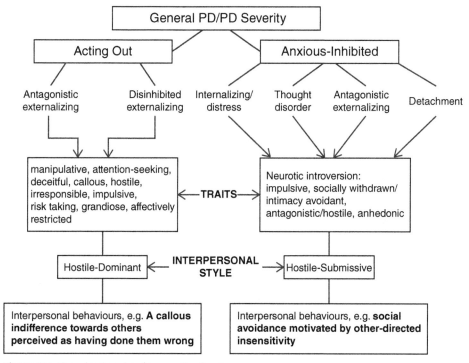

Figure 2.1 Hierarchical model of personality disorder.

characterised by predominantly internalizing features and includes symptoms of avoidant, schizotypal, paranoid and dependent PDs together with internalizing symptoms of borderline PD. It therefore corresponds closely to those PDs shown in the right-hand side of Figure 1.2 as being associated with *maladaptive interpersonal disengagement*.

From Figure 2.1 it may be seen that the antagonism trait *domain* is common to both 'acting out' and 'anxious-inhibited'. However, results of a fine-grained facet-level analysis of antagonism carried out by Sleep and colleagues [27] allows us to see that specific *facets* of antagonism are differently associated with 'acting out' and 'anxious-inhibited'. Antagonism facets of *grandiosity, domineering, manipulation* and *risk–taking* described by Sleep and colleagues are more strongly represented in acting out than in anxious-inhibited. In contrast, the *suspiciousness* facet of antagonism, linked to neuroticism, anxiety/depression, anger and reactive aggression in Sleep and colleagues' results, is a more prominent feature of anxious-inhibited. At the core of both 'acting out' and 'anxious-inhibited' is the *callousness* facet that Sleep and colleagues described as central to antagonism. Both 'acting out' and 'anxious-inhibited' can be considered as variants of antisocial personality, with interpersonal antagonism, callousness and hostility lying at its core.

Narcissism is thought to be a specific manifestation of broader tendencies toward antagonism [28]. While entitlement and self-importance are its core components, narcissism can manifest in grandiose and vulnerable subtypes, reflecting *boldness* (approach-oriented motivation) and *reactivity* (avoidance-oriented motivation), respectively [28]. Grandiose narcissism is associated with a primarily dominant and intrusive interpersonal style combined with low interpersonal distress [29]. It clearly falls within the 'acting out' hierarchy in Figure 2.1. Vulnerable narcissism, in contrast, is associated with anger proneness, suspiciousness, entitlement, self-absorption and interpersonal distress [29]. It clearly falls within the 'anxious-inhibited' hierarchy shown in Figure 2.1.

A considerable advantage of the hierarchical model shown in Figure 2.1 is that it accounts for the emergence of two psychopathy subtypes: a 'secondary' subtype characterised by negative affect, detachment and antagonism together with a *hostile-submissive interpersonal style*, and a 'primary' subtype characterised by boldness, dominance, emotional stability and a *hostile-dominant interpersonal style*. While meanness and disinhibition are factors common to both ASPD and psychopathy, the latter is distinguished by the presence of boldness; psychopathic individuals are not just mean and disinhibited; they can be bold, too.

Interpersonal Style Associated with PD Diagnoses

In a recent meta-analysis of 127 studies, Wilson and colleagues examined associations between PD diagnoses and (1) interpersonal style, defined using the interpersonal circumplex, and (2) functioning in specific relationship domains, including the parent–child, family, peer and romantic domains [30]. Consistent with Blackburn and colleagues' results [26], this meta-analytic review revealed strong associations of ASPD with dominance and coldness and a marked lack of associations with non-dominant warmth and submissiveness. This is consistent with DSM-5 Section 3 criterion A (see Box 1.5 in Chapter 1), which specifies characteristic difficulties in *empathy* (a lack of concern for others' feelings, needs or suffering, and a lack of remorse after hurting or mistreating others) and *intimacy* (an incapacity for mutually intimate relationships, exploitation of others, dominance or intimidation of others). This meta-analytic review revealed clear commonalities in interpersonal style across PDs within the Cluster B PDs (see Box 1.3) whose interpersonal profiles shared characteristics of domineeringness, vindictiveness and intrusiveness. Antisocial, borderline and narcissistic PDs additionally shared a profile characterised by coldness. We might note that several of the PDs examined (paranoid, schizoid, schizotypal, borderline, avoidant, dependent and obsessional-compulsive) shared an interpersonal style characterised by social avoidance. With the exception of histrionic PD, interpersonal vindictiveness and coldness were shared by almost all PDs. In particular, their shared and significant association with vindictiveness speaks to a common tendency toward *distrust and suspicion of others* and an *inability to care about the needs of others*, while their shared coldness reflects an *inability to be generous to and get along with others*. A cold and vindictive interpersonal style likely reflects the high hostility/antagonism that is common to both 'acting out' and 'anxious-inhibited' dimensions in Figure 2.1, while social avoidance is characteristic of 'anxious-inhibited' but not of 'acting out'.

As regards functioning in specific relationship domains, ASPD showed a moderate, significant association with impairment in the peer domain; a modest, significant association with impairment in the family domain; and trivial, non-significant associations with functioning in the parent–child and romantic domains. Effects for the peer domain were larger than for the other relationship domains, and were stronger when assessed using other (vs self) reports of interpersonal functioning and among child/adolescent (vs adult) samples. The moderate association between ASPD and impairment in the peer domain was large among females and significantly smaller, though modest, among males.

Wilson and colleagues comment that, taken together, their results indicate that personality disorders are generally associated with impaired relationship functioning, suggesting construct validity. While they claim that their results support discriminant validity for the different categories of PD, one is more impressed by the commonalities in interpersonal style across the different PDs than by their uniqueness. Results of a study by Girard and colleagues reinforce this impression [31]. These authors examined relationships between interpersonal style and five higher-order personality dimensions: detachment, internalizing, disinhibition/externalizing, dominance and compulsivity. Consistent with Blackburn and colleagues' findings [26], ASPD fell within the vindictive-domineering octant of the interpersonal circumplex (IPC); narcissistic and paranoid PDs also fell largely within this octant. PDs that contributed to the higher-order dominance and disinhibition factors – antisocial, borderline, histrionic, narcissistic and paranoid PDs – appeared to share a domineering, excessively assertive interpersonal style, akin to the hostile/dominant style that characterised Blackburn and colleagues' 'acting out' dimension.

Wright and colleagues subjected the DSM-5 trait model to interpersonal analysis in the framework of the interpersonal circle [32]. Traits related to ASPD were associated with being *domineering, self-serving, and vindictive*. Most traits were associated with interpersonal distress, but traits related to ASPD, psychopathy and narcissistic PD – grandiosity, manipulativeness, attention seeking and risk taking – were *not* so associated. These traits appeared to reflect an interpersonal style marked by being overly agentic (dominating and controlling others) as opposed to feeling as if one is helpless and being subjugated to the will of others.

Summary

The findings reviewed above suggest that differences in interpersonal style do not map easily onto differences in PD diagnosis, suggesting that interpersonal style transcends diagnostic categories. Together with those diagnosed with other PDs that are character-ised by high dominance and high disinhibition (histrionic, narcissistic and paranoid PDs), individuals with ASPD are characterised by a cold, vindictive and dominant interpersonal style that (importantly) does not cause them undue distress. We should note, however, that interpersonal style captures only very general differences in interper-sonal behaviour. We will see in the following section that we have to drill down to a lower level in the hierarchy shown in Figure 2.1 to capture clinically significant differ-ences in particular interpersonal behaviours.

Aggression as an Aspect of Interpersonal Style

We saw in Chapter 1 (see Box 1.2) that irritability and aggressiveness, as indicated by repeated physical fights or assaults, are defining features of ASPD. Recent studies have addressed the question of which trait domains and facets within the alternative (Section 3) DSM-5 model are particularly associated with aggression. In a recent study [33] a nexus of antisocial personality disorder traits (hostility, risk taking and callous-ness) emerged as the most influential facets in driving aggression. However, examination of individual items revealed significant thematic overlap among hostility, risk taking, and callousness traits. Participants who endorsed the item 'I snap at people when they do little things that irritate me' (hostility) also tended to endorse the item 'People would describe me as reckless' (risk taking) – the intercorrelation between these items was high ($r = 0.45$). This suggested a common theme, namely, *a low threshold for engaging in socially directed hostile behaviour*, along with *disregard for others' disapproval*. This same risk-taking item was also more likely to be endorsed alongside the callousness item, 'Being rude and unfriendly is just a part of who I am' ($r = 0.41$), suggesting a tendency toward *negative emotionality that is directed toward others even when unprovoked*. The withdrawal facet within the detachment domain was also found to be associated with aggression. Importantly, significant correlations were found between withdrawal items and items within the hostility and callousness facets. For example, a high correlation was observed between the items 'Most of the time I don't see the point in being friendly' (callousness) and 'I don't deal with people unless I have to' (withdrawal). Likewise, a high correlation was observed between the items 'I get irritated easily by all sorts of things' (hostility) and 'I go out of my way to avoid any kind of group activity' (withdrawal). Similarly, a high correlation was observed between the items 'I get irritated easily by all sorts of things' (hostility) and 'I go out of my way to avoid any kind of group activity' (withdrawal). In summary, three themes emerged, all of which involved patterns of interpersonal behaviour that cut across the domains of hostility, callousness, risk taking and withdrawal: see Box 2.2.

A Role for Motivation in Social Relationships

We noted in the previous chapter that a lack of affective sensitivity, and a failure to affectively engage with others in a prosocial and empathic way, may undermine people's social relationships. We also noted Tyrer's Three I's, prime among which was insensitiv-ity. Antisocial individuals' social interactions are marked by an insensitivity to the interests of others and a preoccupation with their own wants, needs and feelings – they show 'prosocial apathy' to use the term introduced by Lockwood and colleagues [34]. A callous indifference to others is also a core feature of psychopathy [5]. Lockwood and

> **Box 2.2**　Cross-Trait Interpersonal Themes Found in the Study by Dunne et al. 33
> 1. **A callous indifference toward others perceived as having done them wrong** (a high and significant correlation was observed between the hostility item 'I always make sure I get back at people who wrong me' and the callousness item 'I don't see the point in feeling guilty about things I've done that have hurt other people').
> 2. **A tendency toward negative emotionality that is directed toward others even when unprovoked**. The risk-taking item 'People would describe me as reckless' was significantly more likely to be endorsed alongside the callousness item, 'Being rude and unfriendly is just a part of who I am.'
> 3. **Social avoidance motivated by other-directed insensitivity**. A high and significant correlation was observed between the callousness item 'Most of the time I don't see the point in being friendly' and the withdrawal item 'I don't deal with people unless I have to'; likewise between the hostility item 'I get irritated easily by all sorts of things' and the withdrawal item 'I go out of my way to avoid any kind of group activity.'

colleagues pointed to a crucial role for motivation in modulating empathetic experiences. Empathy is not necessarily automatic, but occurs when people are *motivated to empathise*.

A well-established and important characteristic of individuals with high levels of antisocial traits is their tendency to favour short-term relationships and to undervalue long-term, affiliative relationships. Findings reviewed by Mooney and colleagues indicate that individuals who score high on trait psychopathy lack the motivation to form and maintain close relationships with others [35]. Evidence suggests that adults who score high on psychopathic traits, as well as children who score high on callous-unemotional (CU) traits, exhibit impairments in their ability to form meaningful and stable close relationships.

However, it remains unclear *what* motivates psychopathic individuals to engage in social interactions at all. To address this question, Foulkes and colleagues explored what aspects of social reward are associated with psychopathic traits in a large sample of participants [36]. Psychopathic traits were found to be positively correlated with the enjoyment of callous treatment of others and negatively associated with the enjoyment of positive social interactions. The results indicated that individuals with high levels of psychopathic traits may have an inverted pattern of social reward: *they devalue affiliative and prosocial interactions, and instead take pleasure in treating others cruelly*. The most striking result was the strong association between psychopathic traits and what is termed 'negative social potency': being cruel, callous and using others for personal gains, for example, 'I enjoy embarrassing others.' Negative social potency bears a close similarity to facets of meanness in Patrick and colleagues' TPM [13]. Roy and colleagues found that meanness decomposed into two separate facets, *callousness* and *enjoy hurting* [37]. Items in the enjoy-hurting facet contained strong elements of excitement-seeking, for example, *I taunt people just to stir things up; Things are more fun if a little danger is involved.* Roy and colleagues reported a strong association between the enjoy-hurting factor and an overt antisocial factor, in agreement with studies reporting that both affective and antisocial PCL-R psychopathy facets are strong predictors of violence [8, 38]. A recent study examined whether reduced sensitivity to affiliation, conceptualized as a motivational deficit in *responding to, seeking out, or getting pleasure from social closeness with others*, was related to psychopathic traits among 407 adults from the community [39]. Results provided strong evidence that psychopathic traits are related to lower sensitivity to affiliation, and that this lack of sensitivity was specifically related to the affective facet of PCL-R psychopathy and to callous-unemotional traits.

In summary, antisocial individuals have a cold, vindictive and hostile interpersonal style and lack the desire to affiliate with others. However, more information regarding their interpersonal behaviour can be gleaned from specific behavioural themes that cut across traits. An overarching theme is that their interpersonal behaviour is motivated *not* by the enjoyment of interacting with others in an empathic and sensitive way, but rather by the enjoyment derived from harming and controlling others.

A novel approach to investigating the interpersonal behaviour of those with anti-social traits is to enquire of their close associates how the interpersonal behaviour of their antisocial partner or close relative was experienced. For example, a recent study qualita-tively described the interpersonal features of individuals with traits of pathological narcissism *from the perspective of those in a close relationship with them* [40]. Among four clusters of interrelated features identified by the authors was a cluster concerned with a detached connection with others ('emotionally empty') and fostering 'vengeful' and 'exploitative' drives toward others, for example, 'He is degrading to and about anyone who doesn't agree with him and he is very *vengeful* to those who refuse to conform to his desires.'

We saw in Chapter 1 that dysfunctional self-identity and self-directedness were placed together in criterion A of the Section 3 alternative model. We might question what relationship exists between the interpersonal dysfunction in antisocial individuals and deficits in their sense of self. Some authors assume that self-deficits are more fundamental than interpersonal deficits. Clarkin and colleagues, for example, regard 'disturbed interpersonal connections and interactions' as being a *manifestation* of self- and other-representations [41, p. 388], implying that the latter are in some sense more fundamental than the former. Recent findings from a study by Beeney and colleagues [42] suggest that self and interpersonal problems frequently coexist in PD patients and that a complex, reciprocal relationship may exist between them. But *how* interpersonal and self-dysfunction are interlinked is unclear and requires further specification. We employ a model of self developed by McAdams [43] to enquire further into this question, and to enquire how the interpersonal difficulties in antisocial individuals might be related, or even caused by, a dysfunctional self. Below we explicate McAdams' notion that three forms of selfhood – social actor, motivated agent and autobiographical author – emerge in sequence during human development.

Human Selfhood

The self is first and foremost an inherent duality of I and Me [43]. Psychologically speaking, the I/Me dynamic plays out in three different guises: the self as social actor, as motivated agent and as autobiographical author; see Figure 2.2.

Problems in human selfhood as they pertain to psychopathology may be profitably reconceived in terms of the corresponding performative styles expressed by social actors, the motivational agendas of values and goals that energize human striving and determine self-esteem, and the internalized life stories that human beings, as authors of the self, fashion and narrate to make sense of the reconstructed past and imagined future [43].

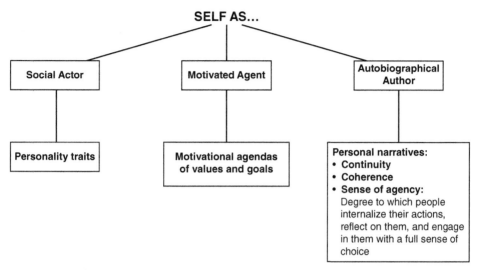

Figure 2.2 McAdams' 'tripartite self' – human as actor, agent and author 43.

Traits are one aspect of the self and are most closely related to the self as social actor. As McAdams states: 'In a phenomenological sense, personality traits are like what the toddler sees when she first beholds herself reflected back in the mirror. The I recognizes the Me.... Yes, that is the kind of person I am, she says. In general, that is how I tend to interact with others and to express my emotion' [43]. Insofar as they endorse the presence in themselves, by self-report, of certain traits and emotions, antisocial individuals clearly see themselves as social actors, albeit their traits and emotions do not conform to a socially accepted standard.

Lykken was at pains to point out that while what he called 'primary' or Cleckley psychopaths were lacking in fear, they were not generally devoid of emotions. He observed in relation to the 'primary' psychopath: 'He seems clearly able to feel anger, satisfaction, delight, self-esteem – indeed, if he did not have such feelings, it seems improbable that he would do many of the things, proper and improper, that he does do' [44, p. 117]. Far from being devoid of emotions, individuals with high levels of psychopathy may experience other-directed negative emotions such as spitefulness and contempt more often and more intensely than other individuals [45]. Given the consistency of their findings involving both spitefulness and contempt, Garofalo and colleagues suggested it is likely that psychopathic individuals experience a range of other-directed negative emotions that involve a *devaluation and derogation of others*. Contempt is considered to be an exclusion emotion [46]; that is to say, its social function is to exclude the other person from one's social network, perhaps because the one who is feeling contempt perceives no way to influence or change the other person or does not wish to change them. If as a result of prosocial apathy one is so disinterested in other people and their feelings or interests, why would one want to change them? From the viewpoint of the psychopathic individual, it would not be worth the effort.

What about the self as motivated agent – in what ways do the antisocial person's goals and values differ from those of most people? We have already referred to the study by

Foulkes and colleagues [36] that provided evidence that the self-serving and cruel social behaviour seen in psychopathy may in part be explained by what these individuals find rewarding, namely, being cruel rather than kind. Excitement seeking is another powerful motivation for antisocial individuals, and as we saw previously (Box 1.1 in Chapter 1), the need for stimulation is a characteristic of PCL-R psychopathy. Lykken [44] pointed out that 'For some people, risk is itself a powerful attraction because it can produce in them an excited "high" that is intensely gratifying.' He further suggested that many forms of criminal behaviour provide this risk-produced high. We will see when we examine sadistic behaviour, in particular, sexual sadism, that the excitement and exhilaration derived from this behaviour is an important emotion goal that motivates it.

What about the narrative self in antisocial individuals? Narrative identity reconstructs the autobiographical past and imagines the future in such a way as to provide a person's life with some degree of unity, purpose and meaning [47]. Unfortunately, we can only speculate about this, since (to our knowledge) it has not been studied in individuals with ASPD or prominent features of psychopathy. Much more research has been devoted to PDs other than ASPD. An example is a study by See and colleagues, who found that adolescents with high levels of schizotypal traits were significantly lower in themes of redemption and agency (agency refers to the degree to which people internalize their actions, reflect on them and engage in them with a full sense of choice) [48]. Comparable studies examining the development of personal narratives in antisocial youth would be a welcome addition to the literature, particularly since, as we will see in the following chapter, adolescence is a critical period for the development of antisocial personality.

Two important points can be made regarding the development of narrative self, according to McAdams and Olson, both of which may hold clues as to what may go awry, developmentally, with antisocial individuals [49]. First, narrative self emerges as a 'first draft' during late childhood and early adolescence. At this stage young people's first efforts at imagining their own life stories may be *unrealistic, grandiose, and somewhat incoherent*; for example, they may hold grandiose fantasies about accomplishment, fame or notoriety in the future. It is only with emerging adulthood that a new and ideally integrative understanding of one's life story comes to be articulated. It is possible that in the case of some antisocial individuals, development is delayed and their narrative self gets, so to speak, stuck at this 'first draft' stage marked by grandiosity, incoherence and lack of realism. This relates to a hypothesis, supported by neurophysiological data, which we will examine in closer detail in the following chapter, namely, that there is a developmental delay or 'maturational lag' in antisocial individuals.

The second point is that according to McAdams the complex interplay between culture and psychological individuality is especially evident in narrative identity – as McAdams and McLean state, 'narrative identity is exquisitely contextualized in culture' [47]. Culture provides each person with an extensive anthology of stories from which the person may draw in the authoring of narrative identity (life-in-culture). A person authors a narrative identity by selectively appropriating and personalizing the stories provided by culture. Stories capture and elaborate on metaphors and images that are especially resonant in a given culture; they distinguish what culture glorifies as good characters and vilifies as bad characters. In America, for example, there are cultural narratives that could support the development of the antisocial personality, from the 'outlaw' in frontier stories to the creative genius who takes pride in his disregard of convention.[1]

Emotions are thought to play an important role in helping to form and maintain cultural identity, reflecting cultural norms and values [50]. People view emotions that fit their cultural model as more desirable. For example, people in individualistic cultures, which emphasize independence and self-achievement, perceive pride as more desirable and guilt as less desirable than individuals in collectivistic cultures, which emphasize interdependence and social harmony. People not only view emotions as more desirable if they support their cultural models; they are also motivated to experience such emotions. They become important *emotion goals* – the emotions people want to achieve when regulating their emotions. Thus, according to Tamir, European Americans ideally want to experience high arousal positive emotions (e.g., excitement), while East Asians ideally want to experience low arousal positive emotions (e.g., calmness) [49].

Dark Traits

So-called dark personality traits are said to reflect a general tendency toward ethically, morally and/or socially questionable behaviour [51]. A 'dark tetrad' comprises psychopathy, narcissism, Machiavellianism and sadism [52]. Key features of this dark tetrad are shown in Figure 2.3. Individuals characterized by dark traits are described as dishonest, cynical, self-aggrandizing, self-absorbed, manipulative and callous [53]. Thus dark personality traits coincide with those shown in Figure 2.1 as being associated with 'acting out', with a hostile/dominant interpersonal style, and – at a higher level in the hierarchy – with a combination of disinhibited and antagonistic externalizing.

A vulnerable variant of dark traits has been proposed comprising lifestyle psychopathic traits, vulnerable narcissism and borderline PD [54]. This vulnerable or neurotic variant of the dark traits construct is likely associated to a greater degree with 'anxious-inhibited' in Figure 2.1. Criminologically, this vulnerable variant has been reported to be associated with drug offences and impulsive property crimes rather than with offences against the person [55].

Although, as shown in Figure 2.3, dark traits overlap in their surface features, their underlying motivations may differ. While individuals with pronounced dark traits may strive for social dominance, their motivations for doing so may differ in emphasis. For narcissistic individuals, establishing social dominance may be a means to gaining the attention and admiration of others or enhancing their status [56]. Psychopathic and Machiavellian individuals, on the other hand, might strive to establish social dominance either as an end in itself or as a means to gratify themselves at the expense of others [53].

Some authors have considered dark traits collectively as a *constellation of antagonism traits*, particularly, callousness and manipulativeness (e.g., [57]). In contrast, Moshagen and colleagues have argued that dark traits extend beyond traits such as antagonism and are underlain by a general factor they call 'D', defined as *a general tendency to maximize one's utility at the expense of others while adopting justifying beliefs* [51]. Otherwise stated, individuals scoring high on D act in a self-interested way to the detriment of others. Gains derived from their selfish action may be tangible (e.g., higher status or monetary rewards) or non-tangible (e.g., feelings of power, superiority, pleasure or joy). Important

---

[1] The authors are grateful to Dr McAdams for this suggestion.

Feature	Narcissism	Machiavellianism	Psychopathy	Sadism
Callousness	++	++	++	++
Impulsivity	+		++	
Manipulation	+	++	++	+
Criminality	+	Only white-collar	++	Sex offending
Grandiosity	++		+	+
Enjoyment of cruelty				++

Figure 2.3 Key features of the dark tetrad, based on Paulhus [52]. Note: A double plus sign indicates high levels of a given trait (top quintile) relative to the average population-wide level. A single plus sign indicates slightly elevated levels (top tertile). A blank entry indicates average levels of a trait.

to note is that Moshagen and colleagues' D includes cognitions, namely, attitudes and beliefs that high-D individuals use to justify their self-serving actions.

Recently, Hilbig and colleagues examined the relationship between this extended dark traits construct (D) and psychopathology [58]. In an eight-month longitudinal study, they found that D, measured using a 22-item scale, was substantially related to all instances of what they refer to as 'socially aversive psychopathology', that is, personality pathology characterised by narcissistic, antisocial/psychopathic, paranoid and – albeit less so – borderline traits. Interestingly, despite paranoia not previously being considered part of the dark traits construct, results confirmed a strong correspondence between D and paranoid psychopathology. A drawback of this study was that it relied solely on self-report measures of personality pathology. Notwithstanding this study's limitation, its importance lies in showing a clear link between personality pathology and dark traits, albeit an extended version thereof (D) that included moral disengagement and spiteful-ness. As the authors state, dark traits and socially aversive psychopathology can be shown to be substantially related once their considerable overlap is represented by D. We will see in the following section that dark traits are strongly implicated in sexual offending, especially in sexual sadism.

Psychopathy in Sexual Offenders

PDs, especially Cluster B PDs, are frequently reported in sex offenders, particularly those who offend against adults (e.g., [59]). Evidence reviewed by Knight and Guay [12] supports the hypothesis that systematic covariation exists between psychopathy and sexual aggression, and that some core components of psychopathy may be inextricably linked to sexual violence and sadistic behaviours. Sexually coercive behaviour tends to be overrepresented among psychopathic offenders, and rapists consistently manifest the highest levels of psychopathy and psychopathy-related traits – particularly the *Machiavellian, callous, narcissistic and impulsive components*, that is, dark traits. These findings are consistently found among both criminal and non-criminal samples.

A recent study addressed the important and understudied issue of the covariates of the severity (vs frequency) of violence in sexual crimes in 302 adult male sex offenders [60]. The PCL-R antisociality facet predicted both types of aggression (sexual and non-sexual), but the affectivity facet uniquely predicted sexual aggression. Borderline traits were prevalent in this sample, with half of the sample having five or more of the standard borderline PD criteria judged present. This underlines the importance of antisocial/borderline comorbidity in violent offending. However, the anger/hostility/impulsivity facets of borderline PD appeared to contribute more to violent behaviour than facets that captured the more internalizing aspects of emotionality.

Sexual Sadism: The Agonistic Continuum

Knight and Guay consider sexual sadism and psychopathy to be distinct but related constructs [12]. Psychopaths and sexual sadists are said to share the following descriptive characteristics: an apparent emotional detachment from the suffering of others, a willingness to inflict harm or pain on another to achieve one's own ends, a desire to control and dominate their victims, an entitlement to do as they please with those whom they victimize and dehumanize, and a lack of remorse about the suffering they inflict on others. Knight and colleagues highlight the importance of 'hypersexuality' for both psychopathy and sadism [61]. A link between hypersexuality and psychopathy was presaged by Lykken, who speculated that a subtype of psychopath ('distempered psycho-path') might comprise men who were at the very high end of the distribution of sex drive intensity [44]. Hypersexuality and sadism have been found to be related both among sex offenders (adult and juvenile) and in the general population [61].

Traditionally, sexual sadism has been viewed as a categorical diagnosis. For example, in DSM-5 it is defined within the paraphilias subgroup as *sexual pleasure and arousal that are rooted in fantasized or actual infliction of psychological or physical suffering on a victim. The fantasies or behaviours must be severe, recurrent, and last for at least 6 months.* Knight and colleagues reject the concept of sexual sadism as a category, suggesting it is more appropriate to think about the degree of sexual sadism (e.g., low, moderate, high) rather than sadistic or non-sadistic individuals. They propose instead an *agonistic continuum*, a dimension that ranges from no coercive fantasies at the low end, through the presence of sexually coercive fantasy and behaviours, and ending in the presence of sadistic and aggressive fantasies and behaviours at the upper end. Recent evidence [62] supports this alternative conception of sexual sadism and suggests that sadism is a progressive disorder that begins with coercive fantasy and graduates into sadistic behaviour; fantasies contribute to early sadism, and behavioural repertoires develop later. The agonistic continuum has been found to be associated with meanness, vindictiveness and narcissism [63].

Knight and Guay's proposed explanatory model emphasises an important distinction between two variants of impulsivity [12]. One variant involves *risk-taking, reward-*

EMOTION ————————→ EMOTION GOAL ————————→ BEHAVIOUR

Feeling bored and unstimulated	Excitement/Thrills	Sadistic violence
Feeling threatened By someone	Self-protection/safety	Violence in self-defence
Feeling greedy and entitled	Self-gratification	Violence to obtain a self-aggrandising goal
Feeling aggrieved, vengefully angry	Vengeance	Retributive violence: to right a wrong

Figure 2.4 Emotions and emotion goals in impulsive and premeditated violence, according to Howard's Quadripartite Violence Typology (QVT). The top two rows refer to impulsive violence, the bottom two rows to premediated violence.

sensation seeking, and disregard for non-goal-related information; the other involves *hypersensitivity to threat, affective dysregulation, and impaired behavioural control in contexts of high negative arousal*. They point out that these two types of impulsivity are not adequately differentiated in current measures of psychopathy. Their proposal is entirely consistent with a typology of violence, the quadripartite violence typology (QVT), proposed by one of the current authors [64]. According to QVT, impulsive violence may be either *appetitively* or *aversively* motivated. In the former case, the terminal value or 'emotion goal' is a desire for *excitement and exhilaration*. When aversively motivated, the emotion goal is *self-protection* from some directly perceived interpersonal threat, physical or psychological.

It is important at this point to distinguish between the *intent* of an aggressive or violent act (to inflict harm on another individual, common to all types of violence) and the goal ('*emotion goal*') of the act. Rosenman and colleagues pointed out some years ago that emotions have distinct goals that guide behaviour [65]. Emotional experiences tend to evoke one of several emotion-linked goals; for example, angry people want to hurt someone or seek revenge, guilty people want to make amends [66]. The emotion goals that operate to drive violent behaviour in QVT are shown in Figure 2.4. Of note is that sexual sadistic violence is driven by a desire for thrills and excitement. This is entirely consistent with Knight and Guay's suggestion that the type of impulsivity marked by risk taking, reward-sensation seeking and disregard for non-goal-related information might be the most important correlate of the agonistic continuum and a key to unlocking the theoretical motivating components of sadism.

Lemay [66] and Knight and Guay [12] both stress an important role for attention. Lemay suggested that shifting attention away from emotions can attenuate the experience of them, while emotional experiences can be heightened by focusing attention on them. Consistent with this, and in keeping with Knight and Guay's proposal, we suggest that when pursuing thrills and excitement, individuals who are mean, vindictive and narcissistic may be particularly adept at shifting their attention away from any negative feelings they may have (e.g., feelings of guilt or remorse). Instead, their attention becomes strongly focused on feelings of excitement and exhilaration (a sort of emotional 'tunnel vision'). Alternatively, when feeling threatened by another (regardless of whether the threat is real) and pursuing an emotion goal of self-protection/safety, they may be so strongly focused on their negative feelings (e.g., feelings of anger) that they are incapable of cognitively reappraising the situation, for example, as non-threatening. This is consistent with the suggestion that individuals with some forms of psychopathology may be insensitive to the *context* in which their emotions occur [67].

A recent study investigated, in two Dutch community samples, whether – and if so, how – emotion goals can be linked to psychopathy [68]. Results suggested that as well as finding anger more useful, psychopathic individuals derive pleasure from experiencing anger – that is, they may *want* to experience it. This is consistent with a typology of anger proposed by one of the current authors that is based on the aforementioned QVT [69]. According to this typology, some anger types, those falling under the rubric of appetitive or 'pleasant anger', are experienced as pleasurable. 'Pleasant anger' was said to be elicited by stimuli that evoke either greed or lust (in the case of coercive/instrumental anger) or that provide an opportunity to maximise positive affect (in the case of thrill-seeking anger). The latter stimuli were suggested to be particularly relevant to the elicitation of anger in psychopathic/antisocial individuals. Results reported in [68] appear to bear this out, insofar as psychopathic individuals appeared to derive pleasure from the experience of anger.

Finally, Longpré and colleagues have outlined several developmental pathways through which sexual sadism might develop [70]. This study indicated different developmental pathways followed by distinct subtypes of sexual sadism. These will be considered in the following chapter, which will consider developmental antecedents of antisociality more broadly.

Concluding Comments

Research reviewed in this chapter points to a key characteristic of antisocial individuals, particularly those with high levels of psychopathic traits, namely, that *they lack the motivation to engage in an empathic way with others*. It is not surprising that these individuals sometimes report that they feel fundamentally disconnected from their social environment. This does not mean that their behaviour is unmotivated or that they fail to engage with other people; on the contrary, it means only that their motives, particularly when engaging with others, are *different* from those of most people, and are viewed by most as deviant. We will expand on this theme in the following two chapters. We also reviewed evidence suggesting that when viewed through the lens of a hierarchical model, antisocial personality, broadly conceived as reflecting an antagonistic and hostile interpersonal style, transcends – and is not limited to –any particular diagnostic category of PD. Antisocial personality is broader than those categories, in particular, psychopathy and ASPD, that have traditionally been associated with antisociality. This is highlighted in the 'dark traits' literature by findings indicating that an expanded 'dark traits' construct – one that includes paranoia, moral disengagement and spitefulness – captures a broad spectrum of personality pathology described by the authors as 'socially aversive psychopathology' [58]. The 'dark traits' construct might be further extended to include *dispositional greed*, a stable permanent personality trait that entails *an insatiable self-centred desire to acquire more resources, coupled with a dissatisfaction of never having enough* [71]. Like other dark traits, dispositional greed has been reported to be significantly correlated with antagonism, egoism and entitlement, suggesting a connection with narcissism [72]. As shown in Figure 2.4, greed – the tendency to indulge in self-gratification, particularly when this is at the expense of others – is proposed to be associated with a specific type of violence that is premeditated and appetitively motivated.

References

1. M. Rutter. Temperament, personality, and personality disorder. *The British Journal of Psychiatry*, 1987; **150**: 443–458.

2. L. Benjamin. Every psychopathology is a gift of love. *Psychotherapy Research* 1993; **3**: 1–24. http://dx.doi.org/10.1080/10503309312331333629.

3. C. J. Hopwood, A. G. C. Wright, E. B. Ansell, A. L. Pincus. The interpersonal core of personality pathology. *Journal of Personality Disorders* 2013; **27**: 270–295. http://dx.doi.org/10.1521/pedi.2013.27.3.270.

4. D. J. Kiesler. The 1982 Interpersonal Circle: A taxonomy for complementarity in human transactions. *Psychological Review* 1983; **90**: 185–214. http://dx.doi.org/10.1037/0033-295X.90.3.185

5. R. D. Hare. *The Hare Psychopathy Checklist – Revised*, 2nd ed. North Tonawanda, NY: Multi-Health Systems, 2003.

6. M. Sellbom, L. E. Drislane. The classification of psychopathy. *Aggression and Violent Behavior* 2020; **59**: 101473.

7. J. M. A. Driessen, K. A. Fantic, J. C. Glennon, C. S. Neumann, A. R. Baskin-Sommers, I. A. Brazil. A comparison of latent profiles in antisocial male offenders. *Journal of Criminal Justice* 2018; **57**: 47–55.

8. S. Krstic, C. S. Neumann, S. Roy, C. A. Robertson, R. A. Knight, R. D. Hare. Using latent variable- and person-centered approaches to examine the role of psychopathic traits in sex offenders. *Personality Disorders* 2018; **9**: 207–216.

9. M. Dargis, M. Koenigs. Personality traits differentiate subgroups of criminal offenders with distinct cognitive, affective, and behavioral profiles. *Criminal Justice and Behavior* 2018; **45**: 984–1007.

10. J. L. Skeem, D. L. L. Polaschek, C. J. Patrick, S. O. Lilienfeld. Psychopathic personality: Bridging the gap between scientific evidence and public policy. *Psychological Science in the Public Interest* 2011; **12**: 95–162.

11. R. Blackburn Psychopathy as a personality construct. In: S. Strack, ed., *Handbook of Personology and Psychopathology*. Hoboken, NJ: John Wiley & Sons, 2005; 271–291.

12. R. A. Knight, J.-P. Guay. The role of psychopathy in sexual coercion against women. In: C. J. Patrick, ed., *Handbook of Psychopathy*, 2nd ed. New York: Guilford Press, 2018; 662–681.

13. C. J. Patrick, D. C. Fowles, R. F. Krueger. Triarchic conceptualization of psychopathy: Developmental origins of disinhibition, boldness and meanness. *Developmental Psychopathology* 2009; **21**: 913–938.

14. R. T. Salekin. Research review: What do we know about psychopathic traits in children? *Journal of Child Psychology and Psychiatry* 2017; **58**: 1180–1200.

15. L. A. Olson-Ayala, C. J. Patrick. Clinical aspects of antisocial personality, disorder and psychopathy. In: W. J. Livesley, R. Larstone, eds., *Handbook of Personality Disorders*. New York: Guilford Press, 2018; 444–458.

16. J. D. Miller, J. Lamkin, J. L. Maples-Keller, D. R. Lynam. Viewing the triarchic model of psychopathy through general personality and expert-based lenses. *Personality Disorders: Theory, Research, and Treatment* 2016; **7**: 247–258.

17. T. O. Paiva, R. Pasion, C. J. Patrick, D. Moreira, P. R. Almeida, F. Barbosa. Further evaluation of the triarchic psychopathy measure: Evidence from community adult and prisoner samples from Portugal. *Psychological Assessment* 2020; **32**: e1–e14.

18. E. D. Gottfried, T. M. Harrop, J. C. Anestis, N. C. Venables, M. Sellbom. An examination of triarchic psychopathy constructs in female offenders. *Journal of Personality Assessment* 2019; **101**: 455–467.

19. R. A. Semel, T. B. Pinsoneault, L. E. Drislane, M. Sellbom. Operationalizing the triarchic model of psychopathy in adolescents using the MMPI-A-RF (restructured form). *Psychological Assessment* 2021; **33**: 311–325.

20. J. D. M. van Dongen, L. E. Drislane, H. Nijman, S. E. Soe-Agnie, H. J. C. van Marle. Further evidence for reliability and validity of the triarchic psychopathy measure in a forensic sample and a community sample. *Journal of Psychopathology and Behavioral Assessment* 2017; **39**: 58–66. doi: 10.1007/s10862-016-9567-5.

21. C. J. Patrick. Psychopathy as masked pathology. In: C. J. Patrick, ed., *Handbook of Psychopathy*, 2nd ed. New York: Guilford Press, 2018; 3–21.

22. D. Yoon, A. Mokros, M. Rettenberger, P. Briken, F. Brunner. Triarchic psychopathy measure: Convergent and discriminant validity in a correctional treatment setting. *Personality Disorders: Theory, Research, and Treatment* 2021. http://dx.doi.org/10.1037/per0000478.

23. M. J. Vitacco, D. S. Kosson. Understanding psychopathy through an evaluation of interpersonal behavior: Testing the factor structure of the interpersonal measure of psychopathy in a large sample of jail detainees. *Psychological Assessment* 2010; **22**: 638–649.

24. S. C. South. Psychopathy as an emergent interpersonal syndrome: What is the function of fearlessness? *Journal of Personality Disorders* 2019; **33**: 633–639.

25. S. Wilson, C. B. Stroud, C. E. Durbin. Interpersonal dysfunction in personality disorders: A meta-analytic review. *Psychological Bulletin* 2017; **143**: 677–734.

26. R. Blackburn, C. Logan, S. J. D. Renwick, J. P. Donnelly. Higher-order dimensions of personality disorder: Hierarchical structure and relationships with the five-factor model, the interpersonal circle, and psychopathy. *Journal of Personality Disorders* 2005; **19**: 597–623.

27. C. E. Sleep, M. L. Crowe, N. T. Carter, D. R. Lynam, J. D. Miller. Uncovering the structure of antagonism. *Personality Disorders: Theory, Research, and Treatment*. 2020; **12**: 300–311. Advance online publication. http://dx.doi.org/10.1037/per0000416.

28. Z. Krizan, A. D. Herlache. The narcissism spectrum model: A synthetic view of narcissistic personality. *Personality and Social Psychology Review* 2018; **22**: 3–31.

29. N. M. Cain, C. Jowers, M. Blanchard, S. Nelson, S. K. Huprich. Examining the interpersonal profiles and nomological network associated with narcissistic grandiosity and narcissistic vulnerability. *Psychopathology* 2021. doi: 10.1159/000510475

30. S. Wilson, C. B. Stroud, C. E. Durbin. Interpersonal dysfunction in personality disorders: A meta-analytic review. *Psychological Bulletin* 2017; **143**: 677–734.

31. J. M. Girard, A. G. C. Wright, J. E. Beeney, S. A. Lazarus, L. N. Scott, S. D. Stepp, P. A. Pilkonis. Interpersonal problems across levels of the psychopathology hierarchy. *Comprehensive Psychiatry* 2017; **79**: 53–69.

32. A. G. C. Wright, A. L. Pincus, C. J. Hopwood, K. M. Thomas, K. E. Markon, R. F. Krueger. An interpersonal analysis of pathological personality traits in DSM-5. *Assessment* 2012; **19**: 263–275.

33. A. L Dunne, C. Lloyd, S. Lee, M. Daffern, Associations between the *Diagnostic and Statistical Manual of Mental Disorders*, Fifth Edition, alternative model of antisocial personality disorder,

psychopathic specifier, and psychopathy-related facets with aggression in a sample of incarcerated males. *Personality Disorders: Theory, Research, and Treatment* 2020; **11**: 108–118.

34. P. L. Lockwood, Y.-S. Ang, M. Husain, M. J. Crockett. Individual differences in empathy are associated with apathy motivation. *Scientific Reports* 2017; **7**: 17293. doi: 10.1038/s41598-017-17415-w.

35. R. Mooney, J. L. Ireland, M. Lewis. Understanding interpersonal relationships and psychopathy. *The Journal of Forensic Psychiatry & Psychology* 2019; **30**: 658–685.

36. L. Foulkes, E. J. McCrory, C. S. Neumann, E. Viding. Inverted social reward: Associations between psychopathic traits and self-report and experimental measures of social reward. *PLoS ONE* 2015; **9**: e106000. doi:10.1371/journal.pone.0106000.

37. S. Roy, C. Vize, K. Uzieblo, J. D. M. van Dongen, J. Miller, D. Lynam, I. Brazil, D. Yoon, A. Mokros, N. S. Gray, R. Snowden, C. S. Neumann. Triarchic or septarchic? Uncovering the Triarchic Psychopathy Measure's (TriPM) structure. *Personality Disorder: Theory, Research and Treatment* 2020. https://doi.org/10.1037/per0000392.

38. M. J. Vitacco, C. S. Neumann, R. L. Jackson. Testing a four-factor model of psychopathy and its association with ethnicity, gender, intelligence, and violence. *Journal of Consulting and Clinical Psychology* 2005; **73**: 466–476.

39. R. Waller, N. Corbett, A. Raine, N. J. Wagner, A. Broussard, D. Edmonds, et al. Reduced sensitivity to affiliation and psychopathic traits. *Personality Disorders: Theory, Research, and Treatment* 2020. Advance online publication. https://doi.org/10.1037/per0000423.

40. N. J. S. Day, M. L. Townsend, B. F. S. Grenyer. Living with pathological narcissism: A qualitative study. *Borderline Personality Disorder and Emotion Dysregulation* 2020; **7**: 19.

41. J. F. Clarkin, W. J. Livesley, K. B. Meehan. Clinical assessment. In: W. J. Livesley, R.

Larstone, eds., *Handbook of Personality Disorders: Theory, Research and Treatment*, 2nd ed. New York: Guilford Press, 2018; 367–393.

42. J. E. Beeney, S. A. Lazarus, M. N. Hallquist, S. D. Stepp, A. G. C. Wright, L. N. Scott, et al. Detecting the presence of a personality disorder using interpersonal and self-dysfunction. *Journal of Personality Disorders* 2018; **32**: 1–20.

43. D. P. McAdams. Psychopathology and the self: Human actors, agents, and authors. *Journal of Personality* 2020; **88**: 146–155.

44. D. T. Lykken. *The Antisocial Personalities.* Hillsdale, NJ: Lawrence Erlbaum, 1995.

45. C. Garofalo, C. S. Neumann, V. Zeigler-Hill, J. R. Meloy. Spiteful and contemptuous: A new look at the emotional experiences related to psychopathy. *Personality Disorders: Theory, Research, and Treatment* 2019; **10**: 173–184.

46. A. H. Fischer, I. J. Roseman Beat them or ban them: The characteristics and social functions of anger and contempt. *Journal of Personality and Social Psychology* 2007; **93**: 103–115.

47. D. McAdams, K. C. McLean. Narrative identity. *Current Directions in Psychological Science* 2013; **22**: 233–238.

48. A. Y. See, T. A. Klimstra, R. L. Shiner, J. J. A. Denissen. Linking narrative identity with schizotypal personality disorder features in adolescents. *Personality Disorders: Theory, Research, and Treatment* 2020: **12**: 182–192.

49. D. P. McAdams, B. D. Olson. Personality development: Continuity and change over the life course. *Annual Review of Psychology* 2010; **61**: 517–542.

50. M. Tamir. Why do people regulate their emotions? A taxonomy of motives in emotion regulation. *Personality and Social Psychology Review* 2016; **20**: 199–222.

51. M. Moshagen, B. E. Hilbig, I. Zettler. The dark core of personality. *Psychological Review* 2018; **125**: 656–688. https://doi.org/10.1037/rev0000111.

52. D. L. Paulhus. Toward a taxonomy of dark personalities. *Current Directions in Psychological Science* 2014; **23**: 421–426.

53. S. Thomaes, E. Brummelman, J. D. Miller, S. O. Lilienfeld. The dark personality and psychopathology: Toward a brighter future. *Journal of Abnormal Psychology* 2017; **126**: 835–842.

54. J. D. Miller, A. Dir, B. Gentile, L. Wilson, L. R. Pryor, W. K. Campbell. Searching for a vulnerable dark triad: Comparing factor 2 psychopathy, vulnerable narcissism, and borderline personality disorder. *Journal of Personality* 2010; **78**: 1529–1564.

55. B. G. Edwards, E. Albertson, E. Verona. Dark and vulnerable personality trait correlates of dimensions of criminal behavior among adult offenders. *Journal of Abnormal Psychology* 2017; **126**: 921–927.

56. V. Zeigler-Hill, J. K. Vrabel, G. A. McCabe, C. A. Cosby, C. K. Traeder, K. A. Hobbs, A. C. Southard. Narcissism and the pursuit of status. *Journal of Personality* 2019; **87**: 310–327.

57. A. Somma, S. B. Vita-Salute, M. Sellbom, K. E. Markon, R. F. Krueger. Assessing dark triad dimensions from the perspective of moral disengagement and DSM-5 alternative model of personality disorder traits. *Personality Disorders: Theory, Research, and Treatment* 2020; **11**: 100–107.

58. B. E. Hilbig, I. Thielmann, S. A. Klein, M. Moshagen, I. Zettler. The dark core of personality and socially aversive psychopathology. *Journal of Personality* 2021; **89**: 216–227.

59. R. Eher, M. Rettenberger, D. Turner. The prevalence of mental disorders in incarcerated contact sexual offenders. *Acta Psychiatrica Scandinavica* 2019; **139**: 572–581.

60. N. Cardona, A. K. Berman, J. E. Sims-Knight, R. A. Knight. Covariates of the severity of aggression in sexual crimes: Psychopathy and borderline characteristics. *Sexual Abuse* 2020; **32**: 154–178.

61. S. Krstic, N. Longpré, R. A. Knight, C. Robertson. Sadism, psychopathy, and sexual offending. In: M. DeLisi, ed., *International Handbook of Psychopathy and Crime*. New York: Routledge, 2019; 351–358.

62. N. Longpré, J. Guay, R. A. Knight, et al. Sadistic offender or sexual sadism? Taxometric evidence for a dimensional structure of sexual sadism. *Archives of Sexual Behavior* 2018; **47**: 403–416.

63. N. Longpré, R. A. Knight, J.-P. Guay. Unpacking the etiology and potential mechanisms underlying the agonistic continuum. Presented at 37th conference of the Association for the Treatment of Sexual Abusers (ATSA), Vancouver, BC, 17–20 October 2018.

64. R. C. Howard. The quest for excitement: A missing link between personality disorder and violence? *Journal of Forensic Psychology and Psychiatry* 2011; **22**: 692–705.

65. I. J. Roseman, C. Wiest, T. S. Swartz. Phenomenology, behaviors, and goals differentiate discrete emotions. *Journal of Personality and Social Psychology* 1994; **67**: 206–221.

66. E. P. Lemay, Effects of emotion on interpersonal behavior: A motivational perspective. In A. S. Fox, R. C. Lapate, A. J. Shackman, R. J. Davidson, eds., *The Nature of Emotion: Fundamental Questions*, 2nd ed. New York: Oxford University Press, 2018; 217–221.

67. Y. Millgram, J. D. Huppert, M. Tamir. Emotion goals in psychopathology: A new perspective on dysfunctional emotion regulation. *Current Directions in Psychological Science* 2020; **29**: 1–6.

68. F. Spantidaki Kyriazi, S. Bogaerts, M. Tamir, J. J. A. Denissen, C. Garofalo. Emotion goals: A missing piece in research on psychopathy and emotion regulation. *Journal of Personality Disorders* 2020; **34**: 488.

69. R. C. Howard. Refining the construct of 'anger' in relation to personality disorders. *Journal of Behavior* 2017; **2**: 1013.

70. N. Longpré, J. P. Guay, R. A. Knight. The developmental antecedents of sexually sadistic behaviours. In J. Proulx et al., eds., *Routledge International Handbook of Sexual Homicide Studies*. Abingdon: Routledge, 2018; 283–302.

71. G. Krekels. Greed. In: V. Zeigler-Hill, T. K. Shackelford, eds., *Encyclopedia of Personality and Individual Differences*. New York: Springer, 2017.

72. G. Krekels, M. Pandelaere. Dispositional greed. *Personality and Individual Differences* 2015; **74**: 225–230.

Chapter 3

Developmental Perspective

The structure of personality (both values and traits) is not as stable as we often assume – the environmental context fundamentally shapes what we are like and how we see ourselves. [1]

The above quotation reminds us that who we are is shaped by our environment, and particularly by the context in which we develop as individuals. We next need to address a hard question: Why is it that, while many people may have personality difficulties, a minority develop a severe and persistent dysfunction of personality that is more or less lifelong and leads them into a pattern of chronic antisocial behaviour? Personality disorder has its origins in childhood and adolescence, as explicitly acknowledged in ICD-11; so for a possible answer to the question of when and why things go awry in those with a severe PD, we need to look at their development during childhood and adolescence. Adolescence may be uniquely consequential in terms of disruptions in personality development, when compared with other stages of development [2].

We saw in the previous chapter that individuals with pronounced dark traits strive for social dominance and tend to exploit others to serve their own goals [3]. Thomaes and colleagues suggested the need for a developmental psychopathology approach to address the question: When, how and why do dark traits emerge? How do they develop over the course of life? And how do developmental changes in dark traits contribute to the emergence and maintenance (vs recovery) of psychopathology? Shiner and Allen suggested some overarching principles of developmental psychopathology [4]. First, study of normal development is critical for understanding pathological development: processes of maladaptation are seen as deviations in normative development. Second, it casts development as an outcome of reciprocal processes unfolding over time; for example, basic dispositions, largely genetically determined, morph into ever more complex personality dispositions throughout childhood. As children mature biologically and encounter a wider range of experiences, the expression of their traits becomes increasingly complex, and this is reflected in the traits they display [5]. The same trait can be manifested in various ways across development; narcissism, for example, may be expressed as grandiose fantasies in childhood, but it may be expressed as concrete status-seeking behaviours in adulthood [3]. Third, psychiatric disorders can best be understood by tracing the pathways leading to, and following from, the development of those disorders. Different pathways and processes may lead to similar outcomes (equifinality) and similar origins may yield a broad range of outcomes (multifinality). Only by better understanding the developmental pathways leading to PDs will we be able to more effectively prevent and treat them [4].

Fourth, a complete understanding of psychological disorders can be achieved only by investigating those disorders at multiple levels of analysis – from biological to individual levels (trait, social-cognitive, narrative) to contextual (family, peers, culture, SES, neighbourhood). The *interaction* of various levels of analysis is important.

Finally, developmental psychopathology accords as much importance to processes of resilience as to processes of risk. Why do some individuals succumb to the effects of environmental adversity, while others survive and may even thrive on them? Relatedly, how and why do some people cease their involvement in criminal activity and manage to abstain from additional illegal behaviours? What are the protective factors that are required to help individuals pursue meaningful and prosocial lives?

Shiner reminds us that the development of personality is closely intertwined with the development of emotions [5]. Although people vary in their temperament-based emotions from the earliest days of life, people's emotional individuality expands over the years to include a broader array of emotion-based traits and typical ways of regulating and making narrative sense of emotional experiences. We saw in the previous chapter that McAdams' self model highlights the fact that people show individual differences in their *personal narratives*, stories about their lives that help them to make sense of their identities over time. We noted that narratives do not become an important aspect of individuals' personality profiles until later in adolescence. Examining the development of life narratives in adolescents with PD symptoms has the potential to yield a richer and more complex understanding of how problematic personality traits emerge during this critical developmental period. Shiner points out that, while many aspects of narratives do not involve emotion, some aspects are emotion-focused [5]. For example, self-defining memories are vivid, strongly emotional specific memories that play a recurring role in individuals' lives [6]. Our earliest memories are often strongly emotional, for example, one of the current author's earliest memories is the announcement over the radio of Josef Stalin's death on the early morning of 5 March 1953, which caused consternation around the family breakfast table.

We will argue that while childhood factors such as a difficult temperament are important in the emergence of PDs, adolescence is a critical period when personality can go awry. Shiner and Allen point out:

> Given that many PDs are characterized by high Neuroticism and low Agreeableness and Conscientiousness, it is not surprising that on average, PD symptoms may peak in early or mid-adolescence and later decline. These findings suggest that the manifestations of PDs may be most intense during the adolescent years, when individuals tend to be the least conscientious and agreeable, and for females, the highest in negative emotionality. [4]

Agreeableness declines with emergence of the child into adolescence, and dark traits such as Machiavellianism show an increase. This is shown in Figure 3.1, taken from a large-scale cross-sectional study by Götz and colleagues [7]. It may be seen that Machiavellianism exhibited a steep and almost linear upward trend from late childhood into adolescence, reaching a peak at age 16. During the transition from adolescence to emerging adulthood, this pattern was reversed as indicated by a continuous downward trend across emerging adulthood, early adulthood and middle adulthood until age 60. It

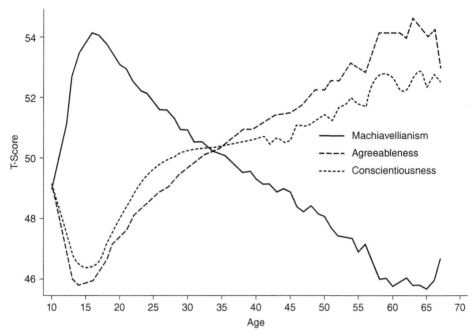

Figure 3.1 Means for Machiavellianism, agreeableness and conscientiousness from age 10 to 67 ($n = 1,117,069$). From Götz et al. [**7**].

may be seen from Figure 3.1 that agreeableness showed a pattern that was the exact mirror image of Machiavellianism, with a 'dip' in agreeableness in early adolescence. A similar dip was reported for *effortful control* in a study of American youth of Mexican origin who were assessed at ages 10–19 [**2**]. The dip was most pronounced for one facet of effortful control, namely, the ability to motivate the self toward a goal when there are competing desires. The dip was exacerbated in youth who experienced more hostility from their parents, associated more with deviant peers, attended more violent schools and experienced more ethnic discrimination, indicating an important role for environmental toxicity in adolescent personality development.

But why do some individuals, a minority, diverge from this pattern, showing a life-course-persistent pattern of antisociality? We will attempt to answer this question in the present chapter.

Sources of Data

Information regarding the life course of antisocial individuals comes from two sources: first, from studies that follow up delinquent youth into their adult years, and second from longitudinal studies that follow up birth cohorts from infancy through adolescence and into adulthood. An example of the first of these is Deviant Children Grown Up study by Lee Robins and colleagues [**8**]. They followed up a sample of 524 individuals who had been referred to a child guidance clinic 30 years previously. These clinic-referred individuals were compared regarding their adult outcomes with those of a control group of 100 children who were not referred to the clinic. Overall the clinic-referred individuals were reported to be more 'maladjusted and emotionally ill' as adults than were the control subjects. Of former patients, 22% met criteria for a diagnosis of 'sociopathic personality' as adults, as compared with 2% of the control group. These criteria included some combination of poor work record history, financial dependency, use of drugs, sexual misconduct and the like. The patients who contributed primarily to the diagnosis of 'sociopathic personality' were those who had been juvenile delinquents as children, but interestingly one third of the 'sociopaths' were judged to have given up much of their deviant activity by the time of the follow-up investigation. This early study demonstrated relative continuity of antisociality from childhood through adulthood, as did another, more recent study by Black [9]. While some individuals were found to improve with advancing age, starting between the mid-30s and early 40s, people with more severe syndromes at onset appeared to be the ones with the most severe ASPD at follow-up. Why some apparently became resilient with age was not clear.

The predictors of later antisocial personality and criminal behaviour are most robustly identified through longitudinal studies that begin with a cohort of individuals who are followed up over time to identify which individuals commit what crimes and what factors explain this. Two of the most influential of these studies are the Dunedin longitudinal study and the Christchurch Health and Development study, both from New Zealand. The Dunedin study reported significant behavioural continuity: children who at age 3 years were characterized as under-controlled (e.g., restless, impulsive, easily distracted) were, at age 21 years, likely to show criminal activity and to meet ASPD criteria [10]. The Dunedin study was able to make an important distinction between those members of the birth cohort (mostly males) who became life-course-persistent (LCP) offenders and those whose antisociality was limited to their adolescence (reviewed by Moffitt [11]). Personality assessments revealed that LCP boys were impulsive, hostile, alienated, suspicious, cynical, callous and cold toward others. As teenagers they self-reported more violence and were more often convicted for violence. By their late 20s LCP men were 2.5 times more likely to have been convicted for adult crime and to be described by informants as having symptoms of ASPD. They self-reported being violent toward partners and children, although few LCP men reared the children they fathered.

The Dunedin study has been able to examine, first, childhood risk factors from birth to age 11; second, developmental trajectories of antisocial behaviour between ages 5 and 26; and third, adult outcomes between ages 26 and 38. Risk factors in life-course-persistent males and adolescence-limited males at different ages are shown in Figure 3.2. It can be seen that the only shared risk factor was delinquent peers in adolescence. Early neurocognitive deficits in the first 5 years of life and childhood behaviours indicative of a difficult temperament were considerably more common in LCP men than in adolescence-limited men. A caveat is in order here. Jolliffe and colleagues reviewed the risk factors associated with LCP, adolescence-limited and late-onset offending based on prospective longitudinal studies [12]. Few specific risk factors were identified that significantly differentiated LCP from adolescence-limited offenders. The authors suggested it may be difficult to prospectively identify who will go on to become an LCP offender and who will have a significantly shorter career and become an adolescence-limited offender. However, the authors' conclusions were limited by the data available to them.

Family Background and Adult Antisociality

As shown in Figure 3.2, several family background factors, including family conflict, inconsistent and harsh parental discipline, and parental conviction were found to be significant risk factors for later antisociality in the Dunedin longitudinal study. Findings regarding the role of family background variables and psychopathy from this and other studies, in particular, the Cambridge Study in Delinquent Development (CSDD), have been comprehensively reviewed by Farrington and Bergstrom [13]. These authors review findings grouped into seven categories: childrearing problems, abuse or neglect, parental conflict and family disruption, large family size, criminal or antisocial parents or siblings, other parental characteristics, and socioeconomic factors.

Farrington and Bergstrom were able to review findings from the CSDD across three generations: the original cohort of 411 boys who were followed up from age 8 to 56, their parents and their offspring. When the original cohort were age 48, they were assessed for psychopathy using an abbreviated form of the PCL-R (PCL:SV) as well as for PD using a structured clinical interview. All three generations were assessed for psychopathy; thus, the CSDD permitted a unique examination of earlier family factors associated with subsequent psychopathy in three generations. In the original male cohort, psychopathy at age 48 was predicted by several family factors: having an uninvolved father, harsh parental discipline and poor supervision, a disrupted family, and a convicted sibling at age 10. Psychopathy at age 48 was also predicted by several socioeconomic factors: low family income, large family size, poor housing, low socioeconomic status and delinquency at school. There were some important gender differences. Compared with the original male cohort, their female offspring showed fewer significant family and socioeconomic predictors. Females compared with males showed lower psychopathy scores and fewer criminal convictions which, in the original male cohort, were associated with higher psychopathy scores (97% of the high PCL:SV scorers received a criminal conviction). Increasing psychopathy scores were associated with a greater number of ASPD symptoms, demonstrating the overlap between ASPD and PCL psychopathy and reinforcing the notion that ASPD and PCL psychopathy are not separate diagnostic entities but instead lie on a single continuum [14]. PCL-R psychopathy scores (total, factor and facet scores) were also found to correlate with total number of ASPD criteria in a German sample of male offenders [15]. In correctional and forensic psychiatric samples, females compared with males are often reported to score lower on psychopathy and ASPD, and to show co-occurring borderline PD [16].

While many of the early psychosocial and family factors have been found to be associated with adult antisociality, Farrington and Bergstrom highlight important methodological problems which prevent easy conclusions being drawn [13]. They point to the importance of sequential effects, for example, socioeconomic and neighbourhood factors leading to family factors which in turn influence child factors, leading ultimately to more offending. The authors point to a pressing need for more research on independent, interactive and sequential effects of family and other factors (biological, psychological and environmental) on the development of psychopathy. A 'cascade' model, outlined in a later section of this chapter, seems appropriate.

Effects of Traumatic Brain Injury

Recently, there has been an increased focus on the effects of early traumatic brain injury (TBI) on later antisocial behaviour. Evidence suggests that TBI is linked to earlier age of

Life-Course Persistent Males

Risk factors (age in years)

	-1.0	-0.5	0	0.5	1.0	1.5
Parents' criminal conviction						
Mother's age at her first birth						
Mother harsh observation (3)						
Harsh discipline (7–9)						
Inconsistent discipline (7–9)						
Family conflict (7–9)						
Mother's mental health (7–11)						
Caregiver changes (birth–11)						
Years single parent (birth–11)						
Family SES (birth–15)						

Child neurocognitive risk factors (age in years)

Neurological abnormality (3)						
Bayley motor test (3)						
Peabody Vocabulary (3)						
Binet IQ (5)						
WISC-R VIQ (7,9,11)						
Reading (7,9,11)						
Neuropsych memory (13)						
Heart rate (7,9,11)						

Child temperament–behaviour risk factors (age in years)

Difficult to mange (2)						
Under control observed (3)						
Hyperactive, parent (5–11)						
Hyperactive, teacher (5–11)						
Fighting, parent (5–11)						
Fighting, teacher (5–11)						
Peer rejection, parent (5–11)						
Peer rejection, teacher (5–11)						

Peer delinquency in adolescence (age in years)

Delinquent peers (13)						
Delinquent peers (18)						

Adolescence-Limited Males

Risk factors (age in years)

	-1.0	-0.5	0	0.5	1.0	1.5
Parents' criminal conviction						
Mother's age at her first birth						
Mother harsh observation (3)						
Harsh discipline (7–9)						
Inconsistent discipline (7–9)						
Family conflict (7–9)						
Mother's mental health (7–11)						
Caregiver changes (birth–11)						
Years single parent (birth–11)						
Family SES (birth–15)						

Child neurocognitive risk factors (age in years)

Neurological abnormality (3)						
Bayley motor test (3)						
Peabody Vocabulary (3)						
Binet IQ (5)						
WISC-R VIQ (7,9,11)						
Reading (7,9,11)						
Neuropsych memory (13)						
Heart rate (7,9,11)						

Child temperament–behaviour risk factors (age in years)

Difficult to mange (2)						
Under control observed (3)						
Hyperactive, parent (5–11)						
Hyperactive, teacher (5–11)						
Fighting, parent (5–11)						
Fighting, teacher (5–11)						
Peer rejection, parent (5–11)						
Peer rejection, teacher (5–11)						

Peer delinquency in adolescence (age in years)

Delinquent peers (13)						
Delinquent peers (18)						

Figure 3.2 A comparison of effect sizes for risk factors for (a) life-course-persistent and (b) adolescence-limited groups, as defined in the Dunedin study. From Moffitt [11].

incarceration, greater violence and more convictions (reviewed in [17]). Life histories of abuse, neglect and trauma are particularly elevated in those with TBI compared with controls, as are ongoing mental health and drug and alcohol problems. Williams and colleagues suggested that TBI could amplify any neuro-cognitive issues due to adverse life events.

As well as noting the link between TBI and early abuse, Williams and colleagues noted the link between TBI and later alcohol/cannabis misuse. This, in turn, might increase the chances of crime. This issue was addressed in a study using data from the Christchurch Health and Development Study [18]. Results of this study demonstrated that TBI during childhood and young adult years was associated with an increased risk for alcohol and drug dependence and engagement in criminal activities and arrests. However, if we focus just on those who sustained very early TBI (1–5 years), several interesting findings emerged. First, they were more likely to show criminality (including violence) in late adolescence and emerging adulthood (18–25 years). Second, they were more likely to show drug and alcohol dependence in emerging adulthood (18–25 years). Third, they showed early-onset substance abuse (in adolescence). Last, and most importantly, the criminality associated with their TBI was entirely accounted for by their adolescent substance abuse. Individuals who in the Christchurch study suffered early (years 1–5) TBI resemble the LCP individuals from the Dunedin study, half of whom were alcohol dependent at age 18.[1] At the very least, early traumatic brain injury would be expected to have exacerbated the neuropsychological deficits (see Figure 3.2) shown by the LCP men in the Dunedin study, albeit these deficits were probably caused in part by toxic environmental influences.

Adolescent Drug and Alcohol Use

Data from the same Christchurch Health and Development Study were used to examine the association between novelty seeking at age 16 (being 'impulsive, exploratory, excitable, disorderly and distractible') and antisociality measured between the ages of 18 and 35 [19]. Higher novelty seeking was associated with unadjusted incidence of all forms of antisocial behaviour, including physical violence toward another, use of a weapon, theft, property damage and dishonest or fraudulent activity. However, after adjustment for alcohol and substance use disorders (assessed from age 18), novelty seeking was no longer associated with any antisocial behaviour. In other words, the effects of novelty seeking on antisocial behaviour were entirely accounted for by the effects of alcohol and substance use disorders. Data from the same longitudinal study showed that adolescent-onset alcohol abuse predicted violent offending both in late adolescence (ages 15–21) and in early adulthood (ages 21–25) even when confounding background and individual factors, including childhood conduct disorder (CD), were controlled [20].

The Jyväskylä Longitudinal Study of Personality and Social Development (JYLS) followed a Finnish sample comprising 196 male and 173 female individuals from age 8 to 50 [21]. LCP offenders were compared with non-offenders, adolescence-limited offenders and late-onset offenders. Results confirmed an early onset of alcohol use (slightly less than age 15) in both LCP and adolescent-limited offenders. Both male and female LCP offenders, compared with other groups, showed greater alcohol-related

---

[1] Personal communication by T. Moffitt.

offending (drunk driving, selling alcohol and detention for intoxication) from ages 15 to 20. Male and female LCP offenders were also drinking more heavily at age 20 compared with non-offenders, and their heavy drinking continued through the adult years to age 50. Results further indicated elevated risk of premature death, persistent poverty and divorce among LCP men.

A recent study used cluster analysis to identify subgroups among 680 young Dutch men aged 18–27 who had been referred for treatment with multiple problems [22]. The following five clusters were identified: (1) 'severe with alcohol and cannabis problems' (4.3%), (2) 'severe with cannabis problems' (25.6%), (3) 'severe without alcohol or drug problems' (33.2%), (4) 'moderate with mental health problems' (22.9%) and (5) 'moderate without mental health problems' (14.0%). The severe group with both alcohol and cannabis problems experienced the greatest amount of childhood trauma and scored significantly higher on psychopathy than both moderate groups. Crime-related outcomes measured at 31 months' follow-up indicated that the severe group with both alcohol and cannabis problems scored significantly higher on most outcomes (violent, sexual, property and 'other' crimes). These findings suggest that there is a significant minority of troubled young men living in the community whose subsequent offending is functionally linked to their past substance abuse.

Together, these studies suggest a cascade of developmental events – from early maltreatment and other forms of family and environmental disadvantage in early childhood, together with TBI in the first 5 years, through impulsive and disorderly behaviour (including novelty seeking) in early adolescence, to early abuse of alcohol in adolescence – as a result of which a career path of antisocial behaviour is entered into. Such a developmental cascade was proposed in a hypothesis originally developed by one of the current authors and recently reviewed [23, 24]. This hypothesis was later elaborated to incorporate the 'dual systems' model of adolescent decision-making and development [25]. Two neural systems, a 'socio-emotional reward system' and a 'cognitive control system', are said to have different developmental trajectories. The socio-emotional reward system reaches maximum strength in early/mid-adolescence and drives adolescent risk taking. The cognitive control system develops more slowly and linearly, becoming stronger through late adolescence and into young adulthood. In reformulating the hypothesis, it was proposed that excessive alcohol use in a proportion of adolescents diagnosed with CD, particularly those showing callous-unemotional (CU) traits, resulted from an over-sensitive socio-emotional system [26]. Critically, this early abuse of alcohol was said to impair and/or delay development of the cognitive control system (and its neural substrates in lateral prefrontal cortex) whose strength increases through adolescence and into early adulthood. Disrupted development of the cognitive control system will then result, during late teens and early twenties, in a chronic inability to control emotional impulses and hence a proneness to engage in antisocial behaviour, including violence. This hypothesis intersects with the idea that antisocial individuals display a delayed cerebral maturation, which we will examine in greater detail in the following chapter. It also connects with the idea that aggressive adolescents are able to disengage morally from their antisocial acts, a process called *moral disengagement* by Bandura [27]. By cognitively framing or rationalizing their antisocial acts, for example, by distorting the consequences of the act or attributing blame to the victim, aggressive adolescents are able to behave in ways that conflict with their values (or with societal values) without experiencing cognitive or emotional distress. Importantly, a study that followed 345 young adults from ages 17 to 25 reported that moral disengagement declined significantly from late adolescence to early adulthood [28]. This suggests that adolescents acquire a greater degree of moral agency as they mature into young adulthood. However, consequent upon disruption or delayed maturation of the cognitive control system, an enhanced sense of moral agency may fail to develop in some individuals as they transition into young adulthood. We return to moral disengagement in the following chapter when we consider the withdrawal or suspension of empathy as an instance of moral disengagement.

How Is Childhood Conduct Disorder Linked to Adult Antisocial Personality and Behaviour?

We saw in Chapter 1 that in DSM-IV/5 the presence of childhood CD is required for a diagnosis of ASPD. Yet estimates of the proportion of individuals with CD who progress to adult ASPD vary widely across samples, from roughly 30% to 60% (on average, the progression rate is probably around 50%). This raises the question of what additional factors need to be present for a CD diagnosis to translate into ASPD. As we have seen above, Howard's hypothesis proposed that the risk of progressing to adult antisociality depends critically on CD occurring conjointly with early alcohol abuse [23]. In support of this, when compared with those showing CD with co-occurring early alcohol abuse or dependence, individuals diagnosed with CD but *without* concurrent alcohol abuse showed significantly fewer lifetime alcohol and adult antisocial problems and, in mentally disordered offenders, less violence in their criminal history [29, 30]. CD symptoms are especially severe when ASPD co-occurs with a borderline PD diagnosis [31], suggesting that greater severity of CD is linked to a more severe form of PD characterized by a combination of antisocial and borderline traits. This is supported by results of a recent prospective study [32] of male Canadian children who were rated at ages 6–12 by their teachers for the presence of conduct problems, callous-unemotional (CU) traits, and anxiety. Conduct problems, regardless of whether they were accompanied by callous traits and/or anxiety, were associated with an increased risk of criminal conviction up to age 24, and of substance dependence, high PCL-R scores and both ASPD and borderline PD at age 33 years. Noteworthy is that risk of being diagnosed with borderline PD in adulthood was increased almost four-fold in those whose conduct problems in childhood co-occurred with both anxiety and CU traits.

Psychopathy in Childhood and Adolescence

There has recently been an increased interest in child psychopathy as a precursor to adult antisocial personality and criminal outcomes. Some studies have focused on 'callous-unemotional' (CU) traits and have reported evidence suggesting that children and adolescents with such traits show a developmental trajectory issuing in more serious and violent offending in adulthood [33]. CU traits have been associated with an earlier onset, more stable pattern and greater risk for antisocial outcomes in adulthood. Results of some studies support the ability of CU traits to predict future antisocial conduct (e.g., [34]), but other studies report contrary findings (e.g., [35]). In the latter study, future violent offending in male adolescents was predicted by self-reported history of aggression, especially physical and reactive aggression, assessed in adolescent offenders immediately following their first arrest. This was the case even when controlling for CU traits, which did not contribute independently to the prediction of arrests for violent offenses. Another recent study emphasised the importance of considering psychological *state*, rather than traits, as an antecedent of offending in adolescents [36]. Scores on the Brief Symptom Inventory (hostility, depression, anxiety, paranoia and psychoticism) were measured at baseline in 1,262 participants, predominantly young men aged between 14 and 18 years who were involved in the American criminal justice system. Raised anxiety, hostility, psychoticism and paranoia at baseline were shown to be significantly related to both violent and non-violent offending assessed 6 months later.

We suggested above that CU traits may be indirectly linked to antisocial outcomes via early drug and alcohol abuse. In one of the few studies to have investigated the relationship between CU traits and substance use, Brennan and colleagues examined the association between antisocial (including CU) traits and both severity of substance use disorder (SUD) and age at which substance use was initiated [37]. They identified two subtypes of SUD-prone individuals, *antisocial only* and *psychopathic*. Their results suggested two separate pathways leading to substance use disorder. A 'psychopathy' pathway, having its origins in CD and CU traits in adolescence, putatively leads to psychopathy in adulthood with the following SUD outcomes: *early* initiation of substance use, greater versatility of substance use, but less severe SUD. It was suggested that the SUDs of psychopathic individuals reflect a callous, fearless, irresponsible disposition that stems from a lack of emotional depth. Interestingly, when the authors used categorical measures of psychopathy and ASPD to analyse their data, a diagnosis of ASPD was significantly associated with earlier use of both alcohol and cannabis. A psychopathy diagnosis, in contrast, was not significantly associated with either outcome. This indicates that ASPD is more strongly associated with substance use than is psychopathy. In contrast to ASPD, psychopathy is associated *only modestly* with substance-related disorders [38]. Of the three components of TriPM outlined in Chapter 2, only disinhibition appears to be associated with substance use (see below).

Lynam proposed that children in whom CD, opposition defiant disorder and attention-deficit hyperactivity disorder co-occurred are beset with a particularly virulent strain of conduct disorder best described as 'fledgling psychopathy' and are at specific risk for later psychopathy [39]. A recent study retrospectively examined whether 'fledgling psychopathy' was associated with subsequent lifetime forensic features, criminal careers and coextensive psychopathology in correctional clients in middle to late adulthood [40]. 'Fledgling psychopathy' was significantly associated with ASPD and to a lesser degree with paranoid PD. 'Fledgling psychopaths' accrued significantly more violent arrest charges for murder, attempted murder, armed robbery and rape/sexual abuse and were much more likely to be chronic offenders. By the time the average client without fledgling psychopathy was first arrested – at nearly age 25 – fledgling psychopaths had an average arrest onset more than a decade earlier. Unfortunately, no information was given regarding early alcohol and drug abuse in the 'fledgling psychopaths', but they may be surmised to have shown a high degree of early alcohol and drug abuse which might have been important in the causation of their later antisocial behaviour.

Dotterer and colleagues investigated concurrent correlates and developmental precursors of the three TriPM components, meanness, boldness and disinhibition, across 17 years of development (ages 3–5 to ages 18–20) [41]. Only boldness showed clear developmental antecedents in infancy and early childhood, including lower reactive control, fewer internalizing traits and greater resiliency. Disinhibition appeared to emerge only in mid-adolescence (ages 15–17) when individuals who scored high on disinhibition showed less prosociality, more externalizing problems, more sensation seeking and more substance use. Disinhibition was distinct from the other TriPM scales in having concurrent correlates indicative of an aggressive and emotionally dysregulated temperament: more externalizing problems and substance use, as well as more internalizing traits. The findings for disinhibition are consistent with the hypothesis that excessive use of alcohol in early/mid-adolescence is a critical factor in the development of adult antisociality.

Dominance and the Pursuit of Power

Another motivational construct relevant to the development of antisociality is dominance or what Johnson and colleagues refer to as the Dominance Behavioural System (DBS; [42]). This is closely related to the dominance axis in the interpersonal circle that we encountered in the previous chapter. Power here refers broadly to the ability to control resources, regardless of whether this is achieved using aggressive, coercive or prosocial strategies. The pursuit of power begins with monitoring cues in the social environment that pose opportunities or threats to the goal of power. Such cues acquire perceptual salience over the course of development. Beginning in preschool, children appraise situations for opportunities to garner material and social resources.

Although the pursuit of power can take prosocial forms, it is related to negative outcomes such as social norm violations, diminished social sensitivity and attention to others, and a diminished compassion for others when they are experiencing distress. In contrast, powerless persons – those who are low on dominance – may over-estimate social threats, such as being disliked or rejected. Johnson and colleagues review evidence suggestive of an association between high levels of dominance motivation and psychopathology. Individuals with narcissistic traits in particular are said to exhibit elevated levels of dominance motivation and behaviour along with inflated self-perceptions of power [42]. High levels of dominance motivation and a diminished compassion for others are characteristics found in a type of sexual sadist that Longpré and colleagues identified among a sample of 518 male sexual offenders [43]. This type, described as 'narcissistic/mean', showed serious conduct problems during adolescence leading to adult sadism. The authors' analyses revealed that offenders on this 'narcissistic/meanness' path had a long history of rule-breaking, which culminated in delusions of grandeur and self-centred behaviour. It was suggested that deficient empathy, pleasure in being cruel to others and a tendency to exploit others are central to this type of sexual sadist. They further suggested that these 'narcissistic/mean' sadistic offenders might set up situations where they can exploit others, and are proactive in their quest for power and domination.

We can relate this concept of dominance and pursuit of power to the 'acting out' versus 'anxious-inhibited' dichotomy presented in Figure 2.1 in the previous chapter. High dominance and the quest for power – particularly when this is at the expense of others – is a characteristic of 'acting out', while low dominance and submissiveness are characteristic of 'anxious-inhibited'. What is not so clear is why and when, in the course of development, the pursuit of power takes on an antisocial expression, but Longpré and colleagues' results suggest that things go awry in adolescence [43]. In the next section we suggest two possible pathways through which antisociality emerges through development.

Gender-Linked Developmental Pathways

As indicated above, one (primarily male) developmental pathway leading to adult antisociality runs from early temperament, psychosocial disadvantage and early brain trauma, through early-onset conduct disorder with callous-unemotional traits in childhood, high novelty seeking and impulsivity in early adolescence, leading to alcohol (and other substance) misuse in mid- to late adolescence. Substance abuse is said to produce deleterious effects on brain development, especially on development of a 'cognitive control' system that develops throughout late adolescence and into early adulthood. We consider neurobehavioural correlates of PD in greater detail in the following chapter.

This 'male' pathway is similar to a developmental trajectory referred to as the 'disinhibition path' by Longpré and colleagues on the basis of their study of 518 male sexual offenders [43]. Having its origins in high school problems, this path was followed by sexual sadists whose offending was characterized by disinhibition resulting from their substance abuse. The authors suggested that as a consequence of their substance use, these sexual sadists are able to maintain their sexual drives in circumstances in which the victim's non-compliance and suffering would normally be sufficient to inhibit them.

This 'male' developmental pathway would be principally associated with the left-hand side of Figure 2.1 shown in the previous chapter. A different (and primarily female) pathway, shown in Figure 3.3, might be expected to lead to the outcomes associated with the right-hand side of Figure 2.1 ('anxious-inhibited') where the predominant traits are those associated with neurotic introversion and the interpersonal style is hostile-submissive. Especially relevant here is Shiner's observation that following the onset of puberty, girls, but not boys, show an increase in neuroticism and negative emotions, changes that seem to continue into adulthood [5]. For some girls, particularly those who score very high on neuroticism and are exposed to intense and chronic interpersonal stress in their early or mid-adolescence, this increase in negative emotionality would be expected to result in behavioural changes marked by social withdrawal and avoidance of

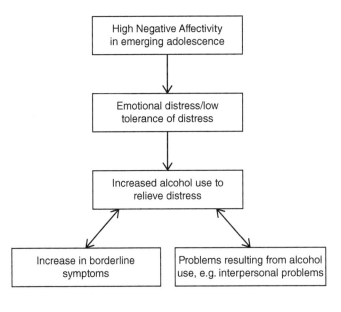

Figure 3.3 A pathway linking negative affectivity in adolescent females to later increases in borderline symptoms and alcohol use. Note: Double-headed arrow indicates that increased alcohol use leads to increased borderline symptomatology, and that borderline symptomatology is associated with concurrent increased alcohol use, as per Lazarus et al. [45].

close interpersonal relationships. These individuals would be distinguished by high levels of emotional distress and signs of disordered thinking, for example, a paranoid distrust of others. Low distress tolerance – an inability to persist in goal-directed activity while experiencing emotional distress – has been found to be a critical factor predisposing to an increased risk for alcohol use and internalizing symptoms in adolescent girls [44]. At the individual level, increased frequency of alcohol use by adolescent girls has been found to prospectively predict an increase in their borderline symptoms, suggesting that alcohol use has a lasting impact on the development of borderline pathology [45]. Moreover, compared with other individuals, borderline patients experience more *problems* when they drink, suggesting they might react differently to alcohol; for example, they may become aggressive or argumentative [46]. Therefore while borderline patients' use of alcohol may be motivated by an attempt to cope with distress, this attempt is likely to backfire, increasing rather than decreasing patients' distress. Although the pathways leading to adolescent alcohol abuse may be different in the case of 'acting out' and 'anxious-inhibited', excessive alcohol use and its harmful effects on adolescent brain development may be a common feature that links both to antisocial outcomes (an example of equifinality).

Concluding Comments

We have seen in this chapter that the route to adult antisociality is marked by a cascade of developmental roadblocks and insults arising during childhood and adolescence. We have emphasised in particular the importance of adolescence as a period when things can go seriously awry and personality can deviate from a normal track. We further emphasised the critical importance of substance abuse, particularly the misuse of alcohol, in the genesis of life-course-persistent antisociality. We have outlined two possible pathways, one predominantly male, the other predominantly female, leading from childhood and adolescence to adult antisociality. One final caveat: we should be cognizant of the interdependence of pathological personality features and disturbed interpersonal behaviour as these emerge during development. Evidence suggests that damaging interpersonal behaviours, for example, being exposed during adolescence to peer-related violence in friendships and in romantic relationships, may disrupt the process of normal personality development [47]. It is unlikely to be the case that personality features unidirectionally cause disturbed interpersonal behaviour, or vice versa. Rather, they are likely to have synergic effects during development, the one potentiating the effects of the other. It is important, too, to consider psychological states (particularly, hostility and paranoia), in addition to personality traits, as precursors of offending in adolescence.

References

1. R. Fischer. *Personality, Values, Culture: An Evolutionary Perspective.* Cambridge: Cambridge University Press, 2017.

2. O. E. Atherton, K. M. Lawson, R. W. Robins. The development of effortful control from late childhood to young adulthood. *Journal of Personality and Social Psychology: Personality Processes and Individual Differences* 2020; 119: 417–456.

3. S. Thomaes, E. Brummelman, J. D. Miller, S. O. Lilienfeld. The dark personality and psychopathology: Toward a brighter future. *Journal of Abnormal Psychology* 2017; 126: 835–842.

4. R. L. Shiner, T. A. Allen. Developmental psychopathology. In: W. J. Livesley, R.

Larstone, eds., *Handbook of Personality Disorders*. New York: Guilford Press, 2018; 309–323.

5. R. L. Shiner. Personality as lasting individual differences in emotions. In: A. S. Fox, R. C. Lapate, A. J. Shackman, R. J. Davidson, eds., *The Nature of Emotion: Fundamental Questions*, 2nd ed. New York: Oxford University Press, 2018; 61–63.

6. D. P. McAdams. *The Art and Science of Personality Development*. New York: Guilford Press, 2015.

7. F. M. Götz, W. Bleidorn, P. J. Rentfrow. Age differences in Machiavellianism across the life span: Evidence from a large-scale cross-sectional study. *Journal of Personality* 2020; **88**: 978–992.

8. L. N. Robins. *Deviant Children Grown Up: A Sociological and Psychiatric Study of Sociopathic Personality*. Baltimore, MD: Williams and Wilkins, 1966.

9. D. W. Black. The natural history of antisocial personality disorder. *Canadian Journal of Psychiatry* 2015; **60**: 309–314.

10. A. Caspi, T. E. Moffitt, D. L. Newman, P. A. Silva. Behavioral observations at age 3 years predict adult psychiatric disorders. Longitudinal evidence from a birth cohort. *Archives of General Psychiatry* 1996; **53**: 1033–1039.

11. T. E. Moffitt. Male antisocial behaviour in adolescence and beyond. *Nature Human Behavior* 2018; **2**: 177–186.

12. D. Jolliffe, D. P. Farrington, A. R. Piquero, R. Loeber, K. G. Hill. Systematic review of early risk factors for life-course-persistent, adolescence-limited, and late-onset offenders in prospective longitudinal studies. *Aggression and Violent Behavior* 2017; **33**: 15–23.

13. D. Farrington, H. Bergstrom. *Family background and psychopathy*. In: C. J. Patrick, ed., *Handbook of Psychopathy*, 2nd ed. New York: Guilford Press, 2018; 354–379.

14. J. Coid, S. Ullrich. Antisocial personality disorder is on a continuum with psychopathy. *Comprehensive Psychiatry* 2010; **51**: 426–433.

15. P. Hollerbach, E. Habermeyer, J. Nitschke, Z. Sünkel, A. Mokros. Construct validity of the German version of the Hare Psychopathy Checklist – Revised. *European Journal of Psychological Assessment* 2020. https://doi.org/10.1027/1015-5759/a000566.

16. V. De Vogel, M. Lancel. Gender differences in the assessment and manifestation of psychopathy: Results from a multicenter study in forensic psychiatric patients. *International Journal of Mental Health* 2016; **15**: 97–110.

17. W. H. Williams, P. Chitsabesan, S. Fazel, T. McMillan, N. Hughes, M. Parsonage, J. Tonks. Traumatic brain injury: A potential cause of violent crime? *Lancet Psychiatry* 2018. doi:10.1016/S2215-0366(18)30062-2.

18. A. McKinlay, J. Corrigan, L. J. Horwood, D. M. Fergusson. Substance abuse and criminal activities following traumatic brain injury in childhood, adolescence, and early adulthood. *Journal of Head Trauma Rehabilitation* 2014; **29**: 498–506.

19. J. Foulds, J. Boden, J. Horwood, R. Mulder. High novelty seeking as a predictor of antisocial behavior in early adulthood. *Personality and Mental Health* 2017; **11**: 256–265.

20. J. E. Wells, L. J. Horwood, D. M. Fergusson. Drinking patterns in mid-adolescence and psychosocial outcomes in late adolescence and early adulthood. *Addiction* 2004; **99**: 1529–1541.

21. L. Pulkkinen, P. Fadjukoff, T. Pitkänen. Persistent offenders and adolescence-limited offenders: Differences in life-courses. *Criminal Behaviour and Mental Health*. 2020; 1–14. https://doi.org/10.1002/cbm.2157.

22. J. Zijlmans, L. van Duin, M. Jorink, R. Marhe, M.-J. A. Luijks, M. Crone, A. Popma, F. Bevaart. Disentangling multiproblem behavior in male young adults: A cluster analysis. *Development and Psychopathology* 2020; 1–11. doi:10.1017/S0954579419001652.

23. R. C. Howard. How is personality disorder linked to dangerousness?

A putative role for early-onset alcohol abuse. *Medical Hypotheses* 2006; **67**: 702–708.

24. R. C. Howard. The link between early adolescent alcohol abuse and adult antisocial behavior: A hypothesis revisited. *SOJ Psychology* 2016; **3**: 1–6.

25. D. Albert, L. Steinberg. Peer influences on adolescent risk behaviour. In M. T. Bardo, R. Milich, D. H. Fishbein, eds., *Inhibitory Control and Drug Abuse Prevention*. New York: Springer, 2011; 211–226.

26. R. Howard, M. McMurran. Alcohol and violence in developmental perspective. In: M. McMurran, ed., *Alcohol-Related Violence: Prevention and Treatment*. Chichester: John Wiley & Sons, 2013; 81–102.

27. A. Bandura. *Social Foundations of Thought and Action: A Social Cognitive Theory*. Englewood Cliffs, NJ: Prentice-Hall, 1986.

28. G. V. Caprara, M. S. Tisak, G. Alessandri, R. G. Fontaine, R. Fida, M. Paciello. The contribution of moral disengagement in mediating individual tendencies toward aggression and violence. *Developmental Psychology* 2014; **50**, 1: 71–85.

29. R. C. Howard, P. R. Finn, J. Gallagher, P. E. Jose. Adolescent-onset alcohol abuse exacerbates the influence of childhood conduct disorder on late adolescent and early adult antisocial behaviour. *Journal of Forensic Psychiatry & Psychology* 2012; **23**: 7–22.

30. N. Khalifa, C. Duggan, J. Lumsden, R. C. Howard. The relationship between childhood conduct disorder and adult antisocial behavior is partially mediated by early onset alcohol abuse. *Personality Disorders: Theory, Research and Treatment* 2012; **3**: 423–432.

31. R. C. Howard, N. Huband, C. Duggan. Adult antisocial syndrome with co-morbid borderline pathology: Association with severe childhood conduct disorder. *Annals of Clinical Psychiatry* 2012; **24**: 127–134.

32. J. M. Bamvita, P. Larm, F. Vitaro, R. Tremblay, G. Côté, S. Hodgins. How do childhood conduct problems, callousness and anxiety relate to later offending and adult mental disorder? *Criminal Behaviour and Mental Health* 2020; 1–17. https://doi.org/10.1002/cbm.2186

33. P. J. Frick, J. V. Ray, L. C. Thornton, R. E. Kahn. Can callous-unemotional traits enhance the understanding, diagnosis, and treatment of serious conduct problems in children and adolescents? A comprehensive review. *Psychological Bulletin* 2014; **140**: 1–57.

34. R. J. McMahon, K. Witkiewitz, J. S. Kotler, et al. Predictive validity of callous-unemotional traits measured in early adolescence with respect to multiple antisocial outcomes. *Journal of Abnormal Psychology* 2010; **119**: 752–763.

35. T. M. Matlasz, P. J. Frick, E. L. Robertson, et al. Does self-report of aggression after first arrest predict future offending and do the forms and functions of aggression matter? *Psychological Assessment* 2020; **32**, 3: 265–276.

36. E. N. Hartsell. The relationship between psychological symptom ratings and crime in juvenile justice system involved young people. *Criminal Behaviour & Mental Health* 2020. doi: 10.1002/cbm.2169.

37. G. M. Brennan, A. M. Stuppy-Sullivan, I. A. Brazil, A. R. Baskin-Sommers. Differentiating patterns of substance misuse by subtypes of antisocial traits in male offenders. *The Journal of Forensic Psychiatry & Psychology* 2017; **28**: 341–356.

38. L. A. Olson-Ayala, C. J. Patrick. Clinical aspects of antisocial personality disorder and psychopathy. In: W. J. Livesley, R. Larstone, eds., *Handbook of Personality Disorders*. New York: Guilford Press, 2018; 444–458.

39. D. R. Lynam. The early identification of chronic offenders: Who is the fledgling psychopath? *Psychological Bulletin* 1996; **120**: 209–234.

40. M. DeLisi, A. J. Drury, M. J. Elbert. Fledgling psychopaths at midlife: Forensic features, criminal careers, and coextensive psychopathology. *Forensic*

Science International: Mind and Law 2020; **1**: 100006.

41. H. L. Dotterer, R. Waller, L. M. Cope, B. M. Hicks, J. T. Niggy, R. A. Zucker, L. W. Hyde. Concurrent and developmental correlates of psychopathic traits using a triarchic psychopathy model approach. *Journal of Abnormal Psychology* 2017; **126**: 859–876.

42. S. L. Johnson, L. J. Leedom, L. Muhtadie. The dominance behavioral system and psychopathology: Evidence from self-report, observational, and biological studies. *Psychological Bulletin* 2012; **138**: 692–743.

43. N. Longpré, J. P. Guay, R. A. Knight. The developmental antecedents of sexually sadistic behaviours. In: J. Proulx, E. Beauregard, A. J. Carter, A. Mokros, R. Darjee, J. James, eds., *Routledge International Handbook of Sexual Homicide Studies*. Abingdon: Routledge, 2018; 283–302.

44. S. B. Daughters, E. K. Reynolds, L. MacPherson, C. W. Kahler, C. K. Danielson, M. Zvolensky, C. W. Lejuez. Distress tolerance and early adolescent externalizing and internalizing symptoms: The moderating role of gender and ethnicity. *Behaviour Research and Therapy* 2009; **47**: 198–205.

45. S. A. Lazarus, J. Beardslee, S. L. Pedersen, S. D. Stepp. A within-person analysis of the association between borderline personality disorder and alcohol use in adolescents. *Journal of Abnormal Child Psychology* 2017; **45**: 1157–1167.

46. E. A. Kaufman, J. Perez, S. Lazarus, S. D. Stepp, S. L. Pedersen. Understanding the association between borderline personality disorder and alcohol-related problems: An examination of drinking motives, impulsivity, and affective instability. *Personality Disorders: Theory, Research, and Treatment* 2019; **11**: 213–221.

47. G. Skabeikyte, R. Barkauskiene. A systematic review of the factors associated with the course of borderline personality disorder symptoms in adolescence. *Borderline Personality Disorder and Emotion Dysregulation* 2021; **8**: 12. https://doi.org/10.1186/s40479-021-00151-z.

Brain and Behaviour Perspective

Livesley argued that a new course needs to be charted in order to gain a proper understanding of PD, one that includes *multiple levels of explanation*, including those concerned with publicly observable phenomena (neurobiology and observable behaviour) [1]. This chapter is not intended as an exhaustive review of the neurobiology of antisocial personality. Its intent, rather, in keeping with the overall perspective of this book, is to focus on brain and behavioural correlates of antisocial personality that inform us about motivational and emotional underpinnings of antisocial personality. For a fuller treatment, the interested reader is referred to Patrick's review of cognitive and emotional processing in psychopathy [2].

Largely driven by advances in brain imaging technologies such as magnetic resonance imaging (MRI), functional MRI and positron emission tomography (PET), recent decades have seen attempts to describe brain correlates of psychopathy and antisocial personality. Some important caveats need to be introduced in relation to these attempts. First, we must beware of a tendency to reduce psychological phenomena to biology, always being cognisant of the fact that PDs are psychological phenomena. Livesley points out that 'Within a multilevel explanatory framework, all levels are necessary for a comprehensive account of PD, and *no single level is more important or fundamental than the rest*' [1, p. 18]. Livesley recommends pluralism as the most relevant philosophical approach, since it recognizes the distinctiveness of each level and the importance of all levels.

Second, we need to pay careful attention to an important distinction highlighted by Ward and colleagues when discussing what constitutes an adequate explanation of criminal behaviour, or antisocial behaviour more broadly [3]. These authors draw an important distinction between an *etiological* explanation, which aims to depict the causal processes that result in a subsequent, downstream effect, and a *compositional* explanation, which aims to describe the mechanistic components that are responsible for the occurrence of a specific phenomenon. Ward and colleagues point out that compositional explanations in neuroscience simply describe psychological phenomena at a different level of analysis; they do not offer etiological explanations for that behaviour [3]. It is important to bear in mind that behaviour cannot be accounted for by simply looking at neural processes. The body, the physical and sociocultural environment, as well as considerations of evolution and development, are vital for understanding both why behaviour is performed, and why it takes the form that it does [4].

Notwithstanding these considerations, a compositional/neuroscience explanation of psychopathology offers three distinct advantages. First, as Ward and colleagues point out, neuroscience methods such as fMRI and event-related potentials generate direct markers of brain activity occurring during a particular task, without the need for the participant to interpret that activity. In other words, brain measures can bypass conscious awareness of the task. Second, a compositional/neuroscience explanation can help in *suggesting* both an etiological (psychological) explanation as well as targets for intervention. With these caveats in mind, we will examine brain/behavioural correlates using different methodologies: resting electroencephalographic (EEG) brain activity and brain event-related potentials (ERPs). Recent (past 10 years) research on EEG correlates of psychopathy have recently been comprehensively reviewed by Clark and colleagues [5]. We will examine brain/behavioural correlates of the three TriPM components – boldness, meanness and disinhibition – to see whether decomposing psychopathy into its component parts and mapping them onto brain and behaviour can improve our understanding of psychopathy as a construct.

EEG Correlates of Antisociality

In a seminal paper, Hill reported a high incidence of what he called 'maturational' EEG abnormalities in psychopaths ('personality disorder with antisocial conduct'; [6]). One must bear in mind that this work predated more recent conceptualisations of psychopathy. These abnormalities all involved an excess of slower rhythms in the EEG and were of four main types: (1) an excess of theta (roughly 4–7 cycles per second) in central and temporal brain areas – this was reported in 19.5% of psychopaths, versus 11% of healthy controls; (2) an 'alpha variant' pattern; (3) focal temporal slow wave (roughly 1–3 cycles per second); and (4) a 'theta dominant' EEG. Hill also reported a higher incidence of posterior temporal slow activity (PTSA) in psychopaths, 14% of whom showed this pattern compared with 2% of healthy controls. PTSA is a maturational EEG phenomenon that occurs normally in children and adolescents. Investigating PTSA in forensic psychiatric patients detained in high security in the United Kingdom, Fenton and colleagues reported a high incidence of such 'maturational' activity in these patients despite their average age of around 30 years [7]. They could find no relationship between PTSA and a range of diagnostic and offence variables or personality measures. They discussed the possible role of early social and environmental factors in the genesis of these EEG anomalies and suggested PTSA may be related to cerebral insult sustained during the early developmental period. In a study by one of the current authors, the EEG records of 265 consecutive admissions to a high-security forensic psychiatric hospital were surveyed [8]. Consistent with Hill's findings, 60% of patients showed anomalous EEG features, mostly an excess of slower EEG rhythms. PTSA was present to a moderate or excessive degree in 55% of EEG records. When the incidence of PTSA was examined in relation to psychopathy in a small subsample of patients who had been assessed using a precursor of the PCL [9], a significant association was found between high psychopathy scores and the presence of prominent or excessive PTSA. No replication of this finding has been reported in the literature. Nonetheless, it is potentially important given, first, findings reviewed in the previous chapter suggesting early brain trauma is linked to later antisocial behaviour and, second, the suggestion that PTSA is linked to delayed cerebral maturation. One possibility that remains unexamined is that early brain trauma is linked to delayed cerebral maturation indexed by prominent PTSA.

Recent studies by Calzada-Reyes and colleagues [10, 11] have analysed the resting EEG in violent offenders using more sophisticated quantitative methods that do not rely on visual inspection. Overall, quantitative EEG analysis showed a pattern of excessive slow wave (theta and delta activity) and decreased alpha activity in right fronto-temporal and left temporo-parietal regions of the brain. These changes were more severe in offenders with an ASPD diagnosis than in those lacking this diagnosis. Using PCL-R to classify offenders as psychopathic or non-psychopathic, and using the same quantitative methodology, these authors reported an increase in fast (beta) activity in the psychopath group, relative to the non-psychopath group, within fronto-temporo-limbic regions [11]. These between-group differences suggested abnormalities in a fronto-temporo-limbic network in psychopathy. Reviewing this and other studies using EEG spectral analysis, Clark and colleagues suggested they lend support to theories of psychopathy that indicate some cognitive dexterity combined with a significant emotional deficit [5].

Neuroimaging Research

Blair and colleagues reviewed neuroimaging research related to psychopathy, considering five broad areas of functioning: empathy, attention, acute threat response, reinforcement-based decision making, and response control [12]. The authors reviewed evidence suggesting that different brain functional systems are involved in each area of functioning. Amygdala dysfunction is implicated in antisocial individuals' deficits in empathy and response to acute threat, but – the authors argue – only empathy is *specifically* impaired in psychopathy. Importantly, these authors suggested two mutually exclusive forms of externalizing behaviour. One form of externalizing, related to empathy deficits and specific to psychopathy, manifests in behaviour marked by *salient callous-unemotional traits and instrumental aggression*. Another form of externalizing is related to an increased acute response to threat and is marked by *heightened anxiety and reactive aggression*. The distinction between these two forms of externalizing disorder is similar to the distinction drawn in Figure 2.1 between 'acting out' and 'anxious-inhibited', suggesting a possible neurobiological substrate for this distinction. At the same time, we should be mindful of the caveat introduced at the beginning of this chapter: a neurobiological description simply re-describes psychological phenomena at a different level of analysis.

An important question concerns whether psychopathic individuals are incapable of activating brain circuits related to empathy or are simply unwilling to do so – they may, as we suggested earlier, simply lack the motivation to empathise with another's distress. Relevant to this question is a study by Meffert and colleagues [13]. These authors studied patterns of brain activation in a sample of psychopathic prison inmates and a healthy control sample under conditions of *spontaneous* versus *instructed* empathy. Participants' brains were scanned while they spontaneously viewed video clips of emotional hand interactions and while *experiencing* similar interactions. Psychopathic prisoners showed deficient brain activation patterns in the spontaneous condition, but importantly, they showed relatively normal activation patterns when instructed to empathise (*to feel with* the actors in the videos). This implies that, as previously suggested [14], psychopathic individuals might be capable of switching empathy on and off at will, depending on their current motivational state. For example, psychopathic individuals may intentionally and wilfully suspend their empathic feelings for another individual when doing so serves their goal of self-gratification at another's expense.

This ability to wilfully suspend empathy exemplifies the phenomenon of *moral disengagement* [15], briefly considered in the preceding chapter. By using self-serving cognitive manoeuvres, aggressive individuals are able to morally distance themselves from their antisocial acts and to *value* violence as a proper means to achieve their goals [16]. Cognitively framing violence as a justifiable means to achieve their emotion goals – excitement, self-protection, vengeance and self-gratification – would allow violent individuals to pursue and achieve these goals without the encumbrance of moral scruples. Results of the Caprara et al. study [16] referred to in the previous chapter suggest that as individuals emerge from adolescence into adulthood they develop a stronger sense of moral agency and hence are less likely to value the use of violence to achieve their personal goals. However, as we indicated, some individuals may fail to make this transition.

Brain Event-Related Potentials (ERPs)

Brain ERPs refer to brain electrical potentials ('brain waves') that either are elicited by discrete environmental events or occur in anticipation of such events. These event-related potentials reflect neural processing on a time scale ranging from milliseconds to seconds. They emerge from the background EEG when electrical activity that is time-locked to the stimuli evoking them is digitally averaged. Since the early ERP studies carried out in the 1970s and 1980s at the Burden Neurological Institute and Broadmoor Hospital in the United Kingdom, there has been a welter of research looking at brain ERP correlates of psychopathy. In their exhaustive review of ERP findings related to psychopathy in the 10 years prior to 2019, Clark and colleagues [5] examined findings in relation to two theoretical models of psychopathy, one emphasizing a cognitive deficit (response modulation deficit) and one emphasizing an affective deficit (lack of fear). Unequivocal support was lacking for either theoretical model, suggesting that an alternative theoretical model might be more appropriate within which to examine ERPs. On the basis of Clark and colleagues' review, it was suggested that individuals with elevated psychopathic traits might be especially adept at screening out distracting threat-related and other irrelevant information, allowing them to allocate attention to stimuli that are goal-relevant (i.e., relevant to their own idiosyncratic goals). The authors highlight that there may be both automatic and *strategic* aspects to the psychopathic individual's information processing, such that those with elevated psychopathic traits *purposefully* spend less time processing distress stimuli. The findings reviewed by the authors suggested that where psychopathic individuals diverge most from those with low levels of these traits is in relation to processing affect-laden content. They highlighted methodological problems in ERP/psychopathy research, in particular, the presence of comorbid conditions such as substance abuse in many psychopathic samples. Research designs that increasingly compare theoretical models will, they suggest, increase knowledge regarding psychopathy. Re-conceptualizing psychopathy using a motivational framework, as suggested in [17], may be useful for designing ERP studies. The role of motivation was highlighted by studies conducted on psychopathic and mentally ill patients detained in high security using the contingent negative variation (CNV) [18]. CNV is a slow brain potential that develops over several seconds between an initial warning signal (S1) and an imperative signal (S2) to which the subject has to make a motor response, typically a button-press. Results of these early studies indicated that when highly motivated, psychopathic patients – particularly those 'primary' psychopaths who were sociable and non-anxious – were able to engage brain processes related to goal-directed action to a high degree.

TPM Correlates

In Chapter 2 the triarchic psychopathy model (TPM)[1] was introduced. In keeping with the triadic orientation toward psychopathy adopted here, in the following section we examine biobehavioural correlates of psychopathy parsed using the TPM model.

Disinhibition

As indicated in Chapter 2, disinhibition (also known as 'externalizing proneness') as conceived in TPM describes a general phenotypic propensity toward impulse control problems entailing a lack of planning and foresight, impaired regulation of affect and urges, insistence on immediate gratification, and deficient behavioural restraint. We noted earlier that according to TPM, disinhibition is a characteristic of numerous disorders and is not sufficient for a diagnosis of psychopathy; this requires that disinhibition be accompanied by emotional detachment in the form of either boldness or meanness [19]. As summarized by Patrick [2], there are two main psychophysiological correlates of disinhibition: first, impaired performance on inhibitory control tasks that generally tap executive functions and, second, reduction in amplitude of the brain P3 response. The P3 is typically elicited in an 'oddball' task by rare or novel stimuli which the experimental subject must detect and respond to. Patrick suggested that P3 reduction might indicate a processing orientation characterized by 'a general tendency to act in response to immediate cues and contingencies rather than on the basis of internal representations of goals and plans' [2, p. 445]. This immediate cue-driven orientation would putatively lead to a proneness to rash decisions, urge-driven acts, angry aggressive behaviour and repetition of past mistakes.

Patrick observed in relation to the development of disinhibition:

> it may be more useful to conceive of externalizing proneness (disinhibition) as an emergent condition of control system dysfunction arising from alternative root sources that operate over the course of development to compromise the formation of frontal regulatory networks … Reduced P3 amplitude may serve as a neural indicator of the impaired elaborative-associative processing that characterizes this emergent condition. [2, p. 431]

This recalls our discussion in the previous chapter where it was suggested that early abuse of alcohol might impair and/or delay development of a *cognitive control system* and its neural substrates in the frontal cortex whose strength increases through late adolescence and into early adulthood. Disrupted development of the cognitive control system would putatively result, during late teens and early twenties, in a chronic inability to control emotional impulses (i.e., to be 'TriPM-disinhibited') and hence in a proneness to engage in antisocial behaviour, including violence. Emerging evidence suggests that the TriPM measure of disinhibition is selectively associated with substance abuse. It shows robust associations with symptom counts for alcohol, cannabis, and other drug-use

---

[1] We use the abbreviation TPM to signify the triarchic psychopathy model, while TriPM signifies the triarchic scales used to measure boldness, meanness and disinhibition.

disorders [20], with more severe substance use symptoms [21] and with poorer substance use outcomes in American military veterans following treatment for their substance use disorder [22].

Disinhibition as conceived in TPM is cognate with a type of impulsivity referred to by one of the current authors as 'emotional impulsiveness' [23]. This has its origins in the work of Shapiro, who regarded impulsiveness as reflecting a failure to control internal emotional impulses and as manifested in affective as well as cognitive and behavioural outputs [24]. A psychophysiological correlate of emotional impulsiveness, both in personality disordered men detained in high-secure care and in community resident men, is the 'go/no-go' contingent negative variation (CNV, referred to above). This is recorded while subjects perform a task in which they are motivated to avoid an unpleasant white noise stimulus, by either emitting (go) or withholding (no-go) a response [25]. The critical measure that correlates with emotional impulsiveness is the difference in CNV amplitude between go and no-go conditions: emotionally impulsive subjects, compared with non-impulsive subjects, show a smaller difference in their CNV comparing go with no-go. This cortical measure of emotional impulsiveness was found to be associated with early-onset alcohol abuse in offenders [26], a finding which gave rise to the hypothesis that early-onset alcohol abuse is linked to the development of adult antisocial personality [27], evidence for which has accrued since its conception and was reviewed in [28]. The cortical (CNV) measure of emotional impulsiveness was also found to be associated with a high risk of both general and violent recidivism in a sample of mentally disordered offenders followed up after their release into the community [29, 30].

Putting together the findings regarding TPM disinhibition and emotional impulsiveness, we can conclude, first, that they reflect a common brain substrate in the frontal cortex that subserves an important executive function , namely, 'cognitive control' or the ability to persist in goal-directed behaviour in the face of competing cognitive and behavioural demands; second, that both arise developmentally through the interaction of pre-existing childhood conduct disorder with subsequent adolescent alcohol (and other substance) abuse; and third, that the impairment of executive function eventuates in rash decision making, urge-driven acts, angry aggressive (and sometimes violent) behaviour, and repetition of past mistakes.

Meanness

There remains a lack of evidence regarding brain/behavioural correlates of the reduced affiliative capacity or 'agentic disaffiliation', seen as central to the meanness facet of psychopathy in TPM. Yet it is precisely the meanness aspect of psychopathy that is considered by many as being at its core [31] and is most crucial for its proper understanding. Meanness signifies the 'pursuit of goals/resources *without concern for the feelings or welfare of others*' [2, p. 443].

Patrick [2] reviewed evidence for a relationship of callous–unemotional traits with reduced fear face recognition and responsiveness, consistent with the idea that the core symptoms of psychopathy reflect a brain-based deficit in sensitivity to distress cues, centred on the amygdala. Additionally, Patrick reviewed findings on brain correlates of pain processing, where the implication is that individuals who score high in meanness would be expected to show differences in brain activity when viewing scenes depicting other people's pain experiences. Findings from neuroimaging studies of brain reactivity to depictions of injury and expressed pain have been equivocal with regard to whether psychopathic individuals show evidence of reduced pain network activation. At the time when Patrick wrote his review, only one study [32] had demonstrated reduced vicarious pain reactivity specifically in relation to the affective or callous-unemotional symptoms of psychopathy.

Boldness

A consistent finding in regard to boldness (also known as fearless dominance) has been its positive association, across diverse samples, with extraversion and its negative association with neuroticism. It is therefore reasonable to assume that the basic personality disposition of bold individuals is toward stable extraversion. Stable extraversion is defined by a dimension running from shy (anxiety and unease in social situations, a lack of social responsiveness) to sociable (liking social interaction) [33, 34]; see Figure 1 in [8]. In the late 1970s and early 1980s, one of the current authors carried out a series of studies of mentally disordered offenders using brain ERPs to examine personality measures in the context of Gray's reinforcement sensitivity theory [35]. Gray's theory posits opposing appetitive and aversive motivational systems that are sensitive to cues signalling reward/ non-punishment (Behavioural Approach System [BAS]) and punishment/non-reward (Behavioural Inhibition System [BIS]) [36]. In agreement with Gray's theory it was found that the shy/sociable dimension reflected sensitivity to cues signalling punishment or non-reward (high BIS sensitivity), with shy/anxious individuals being more sensitive, and sociable/low anxious individuals less sensitive, to these cues (Figure 2 in [7]).

Since TriPM boldness aligns with stable extraversion (Blackburn's shy vs sociable dimension), it too should reflect *a lack of fear*: an insensitivity to cues signalling punishment or non-reward. Three key pieces of evidence support this contention. The first concerns the startle (blink) response that is normally increased under aversive conditions, a phenomenon referred to as 'startle potentiation'. A considerable body of research utilizing the startle modulation paradigm provides consistent and compelling evidence that psychopathy involves reduced sensitivity to threat cues, indicative of a weakness in or heightened threshold for reactivity of the brain's defensive motivational system [2]. Patrick concluded: 'Taken together, these findings point to a contribution of defensive reactivity deficits, linked to a normative individual-difference dimension of fear versus boldness, in psychopathy' [2, p. 436].

Studies with non-offenders (mostly undergraduates) using self-report measures to assess psychopathy have shown reduced threat sensitivity to be selectively related to boldness. For example, Esteller and colleagues showed that diminished startle potentiation was specifically related to boldness in an undergraduate sample [37].

The second key piece of evidence is provided by a study by Ribes-Guardiola and colleagues [38]. They had their participants engage in a card-playing game where they were initially rewarded with money but – across successive trials –were increasingly likely to receive punishment. This enabled the researchers to measure the point at which participants either quit playing (as they were free to do) or continued to play cards. The key finding was that participants with higher levels of boldness (but not higher levels of meanness or disinhibition) tended to persevere with card-playing; that is, they failed to suspend card playing in the face of increasing punishment, and as a consequence earned less money. The lack of restraint in the face of increasing punishment on the part of bold individuals most likely reflected an *absence of fear or insensitivity to punishment cues.*

The third piece of evidence comes from a recent study that tested the hypothesis that psychopathic individuals may enjoy the experience of fear [39]. Participants (under-graduates) were exposed to a fear-inducing video clip and rated their subjective response to the clip as *fearful* (indicating negative affect) versus *excited* (indicating positive affect). Boldness was related both to a lessened negative response to fear-inducing stimuli and to a heightened *positive* response to these stimuli. Not only do bold individuals apparently respond less to fear-arousing stimuli; they appear to interpret (and hence experience) fear-arousing situations as exciting and thrilling. We should note here Patrick's sugges-tion that 'it may be that low fear [i.e., boldness] needs to be accompanied by some degree of disinhibitory liability or callousness to be expressed in maladaptive antisocial ways [2, p. 446]. Supporting this, a recent study found that when conjoined with even low to moderate disinhibition and meanness, high boldness was associated with high levels of antisocial personality pattern and a delinquent predisposition [40].

Patrick further notes that not all psychopathic individuals will show a high degree of disinhibition, which would help to account for the normal executive task performance shown by many such individuals. Consistent with this, and with prior research, executive task performance, indexed by a common executive function (EF) factor that captures covariance across response inhibition, working memory updating and mental set shifting tasks, was found to be inversely related to 'secondary psychopathy' and ASPD, but unrelated to 'primary psychopathy [41]. To measure psychopathy, Friedman and col-leagues used the Levenson Self-Report Psychopathy (LSRP) scales, whose construct validity has been questioned by Sellbom and colleagues [42]. According to these authors the LSRP 'primary' scale does not adequately measure the core affective and interper-sonal features of psychopathy and is most closely associated with measures of interper-sonal antagonism or meanness. Notwithstanding this caveat, Friedman and colleagues' findings [41] imply that deficits in common executive function, reflecting a lack of ability to maintain task goals and to monitor the environment for goal-relevant cues, are unrelated to interpersonal/affective features of psychopathy. A lack of this ability in LSRP 'secondary' (but not LSRP 'primary') psychopaths would arguably lead them to act in irresponsible and impulsive ways to pursue their immediate emotion goals but potentially disadvantage them in the long term [41]. A lack of this ability may addition-ally compromise their ability to monitor the environment for social cues relevant to the appropriateness or otherwise of their own behaviour.

Two Species of the Psychopath Genus: Primary versus Secondary

We suggest that boldness characterizes a type of psychopath who – *in combination with meanness and/or disinhibition* – would have been classed as 'primary' in Blackburn's classification schema, that is, one who is socially responsive, lacks anxiety in social situations and is a stable extravert. This suggestion is consistent with a recent review of psychopathy classification [31]. The authors of this review make a strong argument for a distinction, on both conceptual and empirical grounds, between two main psych-opathy variants: a primary (*bold/emotionally stable*) type and a secondary (*disinhibited/ aggressive*) type, both of which are characterised by high meanness, considered to be the core of psychopathy.

In their review, Sellbom and Drislane point to important treatment implications of this primary versus secondary psychopath distinction. They point out that whereas primary psychopathy is considered largely ego-syntonic, secondary psychopathy is associated with high levels of dysfunctional negative emotions and comorbid internalizing problems. As such, secondary psychopathic individuals may exhibit greater treatment motivation in order to reduce their own suffering. Primary psychopathic individuals are unlikely to find such treatment targets compelling. However, identifying the consequences of their behaviour and the extent to which their choices do or do not support their own self-interests may be more motivationally salient. The authors suggest it will be important to determine whether different forms of treatments (or tailoring of common treatments) are more likely to differentially benefit individuals with different constellations of psychopathic personality traits. We return to this topic when we consider treatment of psychopathy in Chapter 7.

We will see in the following chapter that high rates of comorbidity exist between ASPD and affective disorder. It has been proposed [43] that anhedonia, impulsivity and trait irritability (a defining feature of ASPD in DSM-5) share a common neurobiological substrate, namely, mesolimbic dopaminergic dysfunction, which would arguably help explain the higher-than-expected rates of comorbidity between depression and externalizing disorders such as ASPD.

Summary and Conclusion

In this chapter we have selectively reviewed recent findings regarding brain and behaviour correlates of PD, and of antisocial/psychopathic PD in particular. We noted that one advantage of this brain and behaviour approach is that it provides us with clues regarding aetiology. For example, the finding that a psychophysiological correlate of emotional impulsiveness, a core feature of PD, was related to early alcohol abuse gave rise to the hypothesis that this may be important in the aetiology of adult antisociality. We have arrived at an important conclusion: in keeping with Sellbom and Drislane's review of psychopathy classification [31], we emphasise the distinction between 'primary' and 'secondary' variants of psychopathy, which, in agreement with these authors, we do not regard as a unitary construct. As Sellbom and Drislane remark: 'Psychopathy is not a taxon ... the differences between "psychopathic" and "nonpsychopathic" individuals are of degree, not of kind' [31, p. 2].

This distinction between 'primary' (emotionally stable) and 'secondary' (disinhibited/aggressive) psychopathy variants not only is important for a proper understanding of psychopathy, but also has important implications for treatment, which we return to in Chapter 7 when we consider treatment of psychopathy.

References

1. W. J. Livesley. Conceptual issues. In: W. J. Livesley, R. Larstone, eds., *Handbook of Personality Disorders*. New York: Guilford Press, 2018; 3–24.

2. C. J. Patrick. Cognitive and emotional processing in psychopathy. In: C. J. Patrick, ed., *Handbook of Psychopathy*, 2nd ed. New York: Guilford Press, 2018; 422–455.

3. T. Ward, C. Wilshire, L. Jackson. The contribution of neuroscience to forensic explanation. *Psychology, Crime & Law* 2018; 24: 195–209.

4. K. Nielsen, T. Ward. Towards a new conceptual framework for

psychopathology: Embodiment, enactivism, and embedment. *Theory & Psychology* 2018; 1–23.

5. A. P. Clark, A. P. Bontemps, B. D. Batky, E. K. Watts, R. T. Salekin. Psychopathy and neurodynamic brain functioning: A review of EEG research. *Neuroscience and Biobehavioral Reviews* 2019; **103**: 352–373.

6. D. Hill. EEG in episodic psychotic and psychopathic behavior. *Electroencephalography and Clinical Neurophysiology* 1952; **4**: 419–442.

7. G. W. Fenton, T. G. Tennent, P. B. C. Fenwick, N. Rattray. A study of posterior temporal slow activity in special hospital patients. *Psychological Medicine* 1974; **4**: 181–186.

8. R. C. Howard. The clinical EEG and personality in mentally abnormal offenders. *Psychological Medicine* 1984; **14**: 569–580.

9. R. D. Hare. A research scale for the assessment of psychopathy in criminal populations. *Personality and Individual Differences* 1980; **1**: 111–119.

10. A. Calzada-Reyes, A. Alvarez-Amador, L. Galán-García, M. Valdés-Sosa. Electroencephalographic abnormalities in antisocial personality disorder. *Journal of Forensic and Legal Medicine* 2012; **19**: 29–34.

11. A. Calzada-Reyes, A. Alvarez-Amador, L. Galán-García, M. Valdés-Sosa. EEG abnormalities in psychopath and non-psychopath violent offenders. *Journal of Forensic and Legal Medicine* 2013; **20**: 19–26.

12. R. J. R. Blair, H. Meffert, S. Hwang, S. F. White. Psychopathy and brain function. Insights from neuroimaging research. In: C. J. Patrick, ed., *Handbook of Psychopathy*, 2nd ed. New York: Guilford Press, 2018; 401–421.

13. H. Meffert, V. Gazzola, J. A. den Boer, A. A. J. Bartels, C. Keysers. Reduced spontaneous but relatively normal deliberate vicarious representations in psychopathy. *Brain* 2013; **136**: 2550–2562.

14. R. C. Howard. The quest for excitement: A missing link between personality disorder and violence? *Journal of Forensic Psychology and Psychiatry* 2011; **22**: 692–705.

15. Bandura, A. Social cognitive theory: An agentic perspective. *Annual Review of Psychology*, 2001; **52**: 1–26. doi:10.1146/annurev.psych.52.1.1.

16. G. V. Caprara, M. S. Tisak, G. Alessandri, R. G. Fontaine, R. Fida, M. Paciello. The contribution of moral disengagement in mediating individual tendencies toward aggression and violence. *Developmental Psychology* 2014; **50**: 71–85.

17. L. L. Groat, M. S. Shane. A motivational framework for psychopathy. Toward a reconceptualization of the disorder. *European Psychologist* 2020; **25**: 92–103. https://doi.org/10.1027/1016-9040/a000394.

18. R. C. Howard, G. W. Fenton, P. B. C. Fenwick. The contingent negative variation and antisocial behaviour. *British Journal of Psychiatry* 1984; **144**: 463–474.

19. C. J. Patrick, L. E. Drislane. Triarchic model of psychopathy: Origins, operationalizations, and observed linkages with personality and general psychopathology. *Journal of Personality* 2015; **83**: 627–643.

20. L. D. Nelson, J. Foell. Externalizing proneness and psychopathy. In: C. J. Patrick, ed., *Handbook of Psychopathy*, 2nd ed. New York: Guilford Press, 2018; 127–143.

21. K. J. Joyner, C. B. Bowyer, J. R. Yancey, N. C. Venables, J. Foell, D. A. Worthy, G. Hajcak, B. D. Bartholow, C. J. Patrick. Blunted reward sensitivity and trait disinhibition interact to predict substance use problems. *Clinical Psychological Science* 2019; 1–16.

22. M. Dargis, C. J. Patrick, D. M. Blonigen. Relevance of psychopathic traits to therapeutic processes and outcomes for veterans with substance use disorders.

Personality Disorders: Theory, Research, and Treatment 2021; advance online publication. https://doi.org/10.1037/per0000485.

23. R. C. Howard. Emotional impulsiveness. In: C. Braddon, ed., *Understanding Impulsive Behavior: Assessment, Influences and Gender Differences.* Hauppauge, NY: Nova Science Publishers, 2018; 79–98.

24. D. Shapiro. *Neurotic Styles.* New York: Basic Books, 1965.

25. R. C. Howard. Brain waves, dangerousness and deviant desires. *Journal of Forensic Psychiatry* 2002; **13**: 367–384.

26. L. H. Neo, P. McCullagh, R. C. Howard. An electrocortical correlate of a history of alcohol abuse in criminal offenders. *Psychology, Crime and Law* 2001; **7**: 105–117.

27. R. C. Howard. How is personality disorder linked to dangerousness? A putative role for early-onset alcohol abuse. *Medical Hypotheses* 2006; **67**: 702–708.

28. R. C. Howard. The link between early adolescent alcohol abuse and adult antisocial behaviour: A hypothesis revisited. *SOJ Psychology* 2016; **3**: 1–6.

29. R. C. Howard, J. Lumsden. A neurophysiological predictor of re-offending in special hospital patients. *Criminal Behaviour and Mental Health* 1996; **6**: 147–156.

30. R. C. Howard, J. Lumsden. CNV predicts violent outcomes in patients released from special hospital. *Criminal Behaviour and Mental Health* 1997; **7**: 237–240.

31. M. Sellbom, L. E. Drislane. The classification of psychopathy. *Aggression and Violent Behavior* 2021; **59**: 101473.

32. P. L. Lockwood, C. L. Sebastian, E. J. McCrory, Z. H. Hyde, X. Gu, S. A. De Brito, E. Viding. Association of callous traits with reduced neural response to others' pain in children with conduct problems. *Current Biology* 2013; **23**: 901–905.

33. R. Blackburn. *Personality and the Classification of Psychopathic Disorders. Special Hospitals Research Report, No. 10.* London: Special Hospitals Research Unit, 1974.

34. R. Blackburn. An empirical classification of psychopathic personality. *British Journal of Psychiatry* 1975; **127**: 456–460.

35. R. C. Howard, G. W. Fenton, P. B. C. Fenwick. *Event-Related Brain Potentials in Personality and Psychopathology: A Pavlovian Approach.* Letchworth: John Wiley & Sons, 1982.

36. J. A. Gray. The psychophysiological basis of introversion-extraversion. *Behaviour Research and Therapy* 1970; **8**: 249–266.

37. A. Esteller, R. Poy, J. Molto. Deficient aversive-potentiated startle and the triarchic model of psychopathy: The role of boldness. *Biological Psychology* 2016; **117**: 131–140.

38. P. Ribes-Guardiola, R. Poy, P. Segarra, V. Branchadell, J. Moltó. Response perseveration and the triarchic model of psychopathy in an undergraduate sample. *Personality Disorders: Theory, Research, and Treatment* 2020; **11**: 54–62.

39. A. Book, S. Stark, J. MacEachern, A. Forth, B. Visser, T. Wattam, J. Young, J. Power, J. Roters. In the eye of the beholder: Psychopathy and fear enjoyment. *Journal of Personality* 2020; **88**: 1286–1301.

40. R. A. Semel, T. B. Pinsoneault, L. E. Drislane, M. Sellbom. Operationalizing the triarchic model of psychopathy in adolescents using the MMPI-A-RF (restructured form). *Psychological Assessment* 2021; **33**: 311–325.

41. N. P. Friedman, S. H. Rhee, M. Ross, R. P. Corley, J. K. Hewitt. Genetic and environmental relations of executive functions to antisocial personality disorder symptoms and psychopathy. *International Journal of Psychophysiology* 2021; **163**: 67–78.

42. M. Sellbom, S. O. Lilienfeld, K. A. Fowler, K. L. McCrary. The self-report assessment

of psychopathy. Challenges, pitfalls, and promises. In: C. J. Patrick, ed., *Handbook of Psychopathy*, 2nd ed. New York: Guilford Press, 2018; 211–258.

43. A. Zisner, T. Beauchaine. Neural substrates of trait impulsivity, anhedonia, and irritability: Mechanisms of heterotypic comorbidity between externalizing disorders and unipolar depression. *Development and Psychopathology* 2016; **28**: 1179–1210

The Epidemiology of Antisocial Personality Disorder

It (antisocial personality disorder) occurs and is recognised by every society, no matter what its economic system, and in all eras, showing that it is not purely an indication of a modern 'sick' society. Although its prevalence varies with time and place, the same can be said of almost every psychiatric and non-psychiatric disorder. [1]

Overview

In this chapter we start by briefly summarising the findings from Moran's thorough review of the epidemiology of ASPD published in 1999 [2]. We then proceed to a review of more recent studies undertaken since 2000 to examine the extent to which the findings reviewed by Moran are replicated in the more recent literature. We will address the following questions on the epidemiology of ASPD. First, how common is it? Second, with which other disorders is it associated? Third, what is its impact on psychosocial functioning? Fourth, what is its impact on health services? And last, is its prevalence affected by cultural differences? We end by drawing some conclusions regarding the implications of epidemiological findings, asking what lessons can be learnt from them in terms of aiding a better understanding of ASPD.

Introduction

Problems with interpreting epidemiological data on ASPD exist on several levels. First, a sound epidemiology of PD is predicated on there being a widely accepted nosology. We saw in Chapter 1 that, notwithstanding countless revisions of the DSM and ICD nosologies, problems remain with the classification and assessment of PD, and of ASPD in particular. Should ASPD be regarded as a genuine disorder? The answer to this question surely depends on an adequate definition of 'disorder', but it is far from clear that ASPD refers to anything more than antisocial behaviour and its accompanying traits. A related problem, especially within the DSM criteria for ASPD, is that criminal behaviour is confounded with the psychological traits that are thought to underlie it. This applies equally to the most commonly used measure of psychopathy, the PCL-R, insofar as psychopathy is commonly regarded as a personality disorder. Perhaps the most worrying aspect of all is that the few extant epidemiological studies have all been conducted in advanced Western countries. As a consequence, the twin requirements of representativeness and replication have not been met by the few singleton studies that have been conducted in a limited number of geographical locations.

Epidemiological Studies of ASPD Conducted up to 1999

The role of the health service in providing interventions for personality disordered individuals with criminal and violent behaviour remains controversial. Consequently, the High Security Psychiatric Services Commissioning Board funded a series of studies that might underpin policy. Moran's research was one such investigation. Here, we will do no more than briefly summarise his findings on the epidemiology of ASPD (we might note that he ranged more widely, covering diverse areas such as its natural history, risk factors, etc.). Hence, the following is a synopsis of his findings on the prevalence of ASPD in the community, primary care, psychiatric settings and prisons. Moran observed that despite the heterogeneity of the studies reviewed, evidence was consistent in showing that in the majority of studies the prevalence of ASPD in the community fell between 2 and 3% of the population sampled [2]. He also identified that single young men who were poorly educated and impoverished were particularly vulnerable. While in primary care, the prevalence rate for attendees varied between 5 and 11%; this diminished in psychiatric settings where unselected admissions showed a low prevalence rate of 1–3%. The data from high-secure hospitals in England and Wales were compromised by the use, in almost all studies, of the legal designation 'psychopathic disorder' rather than by an operationally defined clinical diagnosis. An exception was a study that applied the criteria of the Structured Clinical Interview for DSM-IV Axis II Personality Disorders (SCID-II) to legally define 'psychopaths' and found rates of 38% and 44% for ASPD in men and women, respectively [3]. Finally, Moran concluded that the rate of ASPD in prisons was between 40 and 60%, though he noted that this area was fraught with methodological problems. He also observed that ASPD frequently occurred comorbidly with other mental illnesses and with other personality disorders, especially borderline, narcissistic and paranoid PDs. He observed that ASPD placed considerable burden on both the sufferer and those around him. Moran was at pains to point out that many of the studies on which his report was based were methodologically flawed. This particularly applied to community studies as none of these were properly representative of the entire population. For instance, where 'normal control' samples were used, these were usually community volunteers matched to the host sample.

Torgersen and colleagues provided a helpful summary of 10 community studies conducted between 1989 and 1998 [4]. This showed pooled averages of 13.5% and 1.6% for any personality disorder and for ASPD, respectively. In an updated review published in 2012 he included six studies published in the early 2000s. These showed a range of 3.9–14.3% and a median of 11.9% for any personality disorder. For ASPD, the range was 0.2–4.5% with a median of 1.0% [5].

Epidemiological Studies of ASPD since 2000

The turn of the century represented a sea-change in methodological rigour in investigating the prevalence of personality disorder (including ASPD) in the community. Latterly, the studies have been methodologically superior, being larger, evaluating more representative samples, using accepted diagnostic instruments and applying statistical rigour to the results. We will address the question of whether these more methodologically sophisticated studies produced findings that were any different from their predecessors. We have chosen eight of these major studies, which, as might be anticipated, vary in both their design and results. It is nonetheless instructive to compare these studies with one another. We summarise the design, the assessments used, and the results from each of these studies in chronological order in Table 5.1; a summary is presented in Table 5.2. In keeping with the purposes of an epidemiological inquiry into ASPD outlined above, the studies chosen ought to enable us to update our knowledge on the following questions in respect of ASPD: (1) its prevalence, (2) its comorbidity, (3) its impact on psychosocial adjustment, (4) its impact on health services and (5) its cross-cultural variation. We consider these in turn below.

We should note that although all studies claim to be representative of the population from which the sample was drawn, only the NESARC [6] and Coid et al. [7] studies truly meet the criteria for being nationally representative. They also have varying sizes, from 626 in Coid et al. [7] to the 43,093 in Grant et al.'s study [6] and 36,309 in Goldstein et al.'s study [8]. A major limitation of all the studies was their exclusively Western perspective, since they were based on samples either from the United States (six studies) or Europe (two studies). While the results from the International Personality Disorder Examination field trial suggest that the majority of personality disorder subtypes can be diagnosed in most countries [9], this was only a single study that was not intended as an epidemiological investigation. Hence, with the exception of Goldstein and colleagues' investigation [8], we have very few data that reported on the cross-cultural variation of personality disorder in general and of ASPD in particular.

Prevalence Rates

The prevalence rates for any personality disorder in these selected studies ranged from 4.4% [7] to 21.5% [6]. For ASPD, the range was 0.6% [7] to 4.3% [8]. All of the studies used the Diagnostic Statistical Manuel (DSM) definitions of PD (with varying criteria from DSM-III to DSM-5) with the exception of the Samuels and colleagues' study [10]. This used the IPDE to assess the same individuals using DSM-IV ASPD and ICD-10 Dissocial PD criteria, reporting prevalence rates of 4.1% and 3%, respectively.

There are a number of possible reasons for these differences in reported rates for ASPD. The first has to do with differences in the mode of assessment. For instance, some studies (e.g., the first publication from the NESARC study [6]) employed lay assessors using a non-validated instrument (i.e., the Alcohol Use Disorder and Associated Disabilities Interview Schedule – DSM-IV Version (AUDADIS) for PD with the requirement that 'at least one positive symptom item (of PD) must have caused social or occupational dysfunction' [6, p. 363]. When Trull and colleagues applied a more stringent criterion, namely, that each personality disorder criterion be associated with distress/impairment in order to count toward a diagnosis, the prevalence for any PD fell from 21.5% to 9.1%, although the prevalence of ASPD remained the same, 3.8% [11]. The second reason for the different prevalence rates is that the two studies conducted in Europe reported very low prevalences of ASPD (0.6% and 0.7%). This contrasts with a far higher prevalence (3.5%) of ASPD reported by the six studies carried out in the United States. It has been suggested that that the higher rates of ASPD in the United States might reflect cultural differences, which we consider below. A third possible reason for the differing prevalence rates is that some studies focused solely on an urban environment rather than being nationally representative (e.g., [5]). As a consequence, these studies yielded higher prevalence rates since ASPD is noted to be more common in urban settings (8). Notable in this context is that Torgersen and colleagues studied individuals

Table 5.1 Study design and results of eight studies conducted between 2000 and 2017

Study	Design and sample	Size of sample	Diagnostic instrument(s) used	Weighted prevalence rates of any PD and ASPD	Rates of ASPD in males and females	Comorbidity studied
Torgensen et al. (2001)	Representative sample from one urban area (i.e., Oslo, Norway)	n = 2,053	Structural Interview for DSM-III-R (SIPD-R) for PD	Any PD = 13.8% ASPD = 0.7%	Males = 0.7% Females = 0.0%	No
Samuels et al. (2003)	Representative sample from the Baltimore Epidemiological Catchment Area Study (US)	n = 742	IPDE interviewer by trained interviewers who also interviewed an informant – both DSM-IV and ICD-10 reported on	Any PD = 9% (DSM) 5.0 (ICD) ASPD = 4.1% Dissocial PD = 3%	Not reported formally but younger males had the greatest association with ASPD	Axis I conditions not studied but socio-demographics were considered
Grant et al. (2004)	National representative sample from the US	n = 43,093	AUDADIS-IV Direct interview to determine association between alcohol and drug use with seven DSM-IV PDs. Lay interviewers face to face.	12-month prevalence of any PD = 14.5%; of ASPD = 3.6%	Not reported	12-month prevalence for any PD comorbid with alcohol use disorder = 16.3%; for ASPD = 28.7%. For drug use disorder any PD = 6.5%; for ASPD = 15.2%
Crawford et al. (2005)	Follow-up of a nationally representative sample (i.e., Children in the Community) (US). Subjects had a mean age of 33.	n = 644	CIS-SR (i.e, a self-report instrument) and SCID-11 (by direct interview)	Any PD at age 22 = 11.2% (CIS-SR) and 15.7% (SCID-11) ASPD = 2.3% (CIS-SR) and 1.2% (SCID)	Not reported	Disability measured by psychosocial impairment and global assessment of functioning (GAF)

Study	Description	n	Assessment	Prevalence	Sex prevalence	Comorbidity
Coid et al. (2006)	Representative sample from the general population in Scotland, England and Wales	n = 626	SCID-11 interview by trained interviewers and SCAN, CIS-R and AUDIT for Axis I conditions	Any PD = 4.4% ASPD = 0.6%	Males = 1.0% Females = 0.2%	Axis I conditions studied
Lenzenweger et al. (2007)	National Comorbidity Survey – Replication (NCS-R) (US)	n = 5,692	IPDE Interviewed by trained interviewers on subsample n = 214 using DSM-IV	Any PD = 9.1% ASPD = 0.6% or = 1% in the clinical reappraisal sample	Not reported	Axis I conditions studied
Trull et al. (2010)	Re-analysis of the NESARC data using stricter criteria (US)	n = 43,093	AUDADIS-IV Direct interview with lay interviewers	Any PD = 9.1% ASPD = 3.8%	Males = 5.5% Females = 1.9%	Comorbidity assessed as per the NESARC schedule
Goldstein et al. (2017)	Analysis of NESARC –III data using DSM-5 PD criteria (US)	n = 36,309	ADUADIS-V Direct interview with lay interviewers	ASPD = 4.3%	Odds ratio male and female = 3.5.	Comorbidity assessed as per NESCARC schedule

Table 5.2 Summary of prevalence rates of any PD and of ASPD among the eight studies examined

Study	Prevalence of any PD (%)	Prevalence of ASPD (%)
Torgensen et al. (2001)	13.8	0.7
Samuels et al. (2003)	9	4.1
Grant et al. (2004)	14.5[a] and 21.5[b]	3.6
Crawford et al. (2005)	13.4	1.7
Coid et al. (2006)	4.4[c]	0.6
Lenzenweger et al. (2007)	9.1	1
Trull et al. (2010)	9.1	3.6
Goldstein et al. (2017)	-	4.3

[a] Data from Wave 1 of the NESCAR study when three personality disorders were excluded.
[b] Prevalence from Wave 2 when these are included and combined with Wave 1.
[c] Weighted prevalence.

in a European urban environment and yet found a prevalence of only 0.7% [4, 5]. It is likely that the increased prevalence of ASPD in the US studies is a consequence of both methodological and cultural differences between the United States and Europe. Despite the methodological differences in sampling, method of assessment and statistical adjustment, the mean prevalence of ASPD across these eight studies is 2.45%, a figure that is similar to those (2–3%) reported by Moran [2]. However, for the reasons outlined above the prevalence of ASPD in European populations is likely to be close to 1% or even lower.

Gender Differences

One of the most striking and consistent findings in the epidemiological literature on ASPD is its marked difference in prevalence, with a gender ratio of 3:1 for men and women. For instance, Robins and Regier, reporting on the Epidemiological Catchment Area Survey, found that 2–4% of men and 0.5–1% of women fulfilled DSM-III-R criteria for ASPD [12]. While the prevalence rates were lower in the two European studies, similar differences between men and women were found with rates of 1% in men and 0% in women in [4], 1.3% in men and 0.2% in [7]. As ever in epidemiological inquiries, this difference raises an important question: Is this a real difference or a methodological artefact? This has been usefully explored by Bishop and colleagues in a review [13] where they argue that the inclusion of conduct disorder as a necessary condition for the diagnosis of ASPD in adulthood is problematic in estimating the prevalence of ASPD in adult women. This is because conduct disorder presents later in girls than boys and shows a marked difference in its presentation: boys were found to be overall more physically aggressive, impulsive and to exhibit more externalizing behaviours, whereas girls were more anxious, likely to run away from home and exhibit more internalizing behaviours [14]. Anxiety was the only positive predictor found for girls with conduct disorder who subsequently developed ASPD [14]. Antisocial behaviour in later life therefore appears to be underpinned by a greater vulnerability to stress and emotional dysregulation in women in contrast to the callousness or lack of empathy seen in men [14]. This is supported by work on adverse life events where adult women suffer emotional abuse, sexual abuse and physical abuse [15]. These epidemiological differences clearly have implications, not only for our understanding of the aetiology of ASPD (see Chapter 3) but also for treatment, discussed further in Chapter 6.

Comorbidity of ASPD with Psychiatric Syndromes

Several of the studies reported on the comorbidity between PD and other mental illnesses and with other personality disorders. Coid and colleagues [7] provided the most thorough assessment of any co-occurring mental illnesses as their study was the only one to provide an assessment of psychotic disorders. Unfortunately, their results were presented by cluster rather than by individual personality disorder. Nonetheless, they reported that compared with Clusters A and C, the highest associations for Cluster B PDs were with a functional psychosis (odds ratio [OR] = 7.44) and an affective/anxiety disorder (OR = 20.3) [7]. Lenzenweger and colleagues again found that while all three clusters were associated with mental illnesses, the strongest association was with Cluster B disorders [16]. Reporting on two individual personality disorders (ASPD and borderline PD), this study found that 70% of those with ASPD met criteria for at least one 12-month mental illness with an average of 3.4 disorders. Goldstein and colleagues [8] reported that among those with ASPD, the lifetime prevalences for any mood disorder and any anxiety disorder were 51.5% and 35.8%, respectively. While many of the studies found an association between ASPD and substance misuse, the NESARC studies [6, 8, 11] had a primary focus on this area. In summary, high rates of comorbidity between substance misuse and any PD were reported in all three investigations, but the rates were highest for those with ASPD. For example, while 12-month prevalence rates of alcohol use disorder (AUD) and drug use disorder (DUD) were 16.4% and 6.5%, respectively, for those with any PD, for those with ASPD these rose to 28.7% and 15.2%, respectively [6]. Another study investigated past year DUD and AUD in the NESARC-III sample but separately in those with just ASPD and those who showed ASPD comorbidly with borderline PD [17]. Prevalence of AUD (39.4%) and DUD (22.6%) was especially high in those who showed ASPD comorbidly with borderline PD compared with those who showed ASPD alone (31.2% and 10.5%, respectively). Those who showed neither ASPD nor borderline PD showed substantially lower prevalences: 11.2% for AUD and 2.3% for DUD. It is noteworthy that the prevalence of antisocial/borderline PD comorbidity in this US sample was high (2.2%) compared with that reported for the United Kingdom (0.3% [7]).

Comorbidity of ASPD with Other Personality Disorders

We turn, finally, to the comorbidity of ASPD with other personality disorders. This is a contentious area, with some arguing that these are not true comorbidities, but rather are an inevitable artefact of the categorical classification of personality disorder [18, 19]. We should therefore rather talk of *co-occurrence* of PDs than of comorbidity. Indeed the high 'comorbidity' between PDs is one of the major reasons why revisions of the current system are deemed to be necessary [20]. Putting this objection to one side, we will restrict ourselves to a few brief comments. The current data can be summarised as follows:

1. The co-occurrence of ASPD with other personality disorders is relatively uncommon, being lower than among all other personality disorders [21]. However, an important caveat here is that, as Trull and colleagues pointed out, 'one's evaluation of how

highly associated or comorbid a PD is with other PDs seems to vary, (sometimes dramatically) depending on the sample ... an important distinction seems to be whether one is examining comorbidity in the general population or in clinical samples' [21, p. 229].

2. When it does occur, comorbidity of ASPD is largely with other Cluster B disorders (especially borderline and narcissistic PDs) and with paranoid PD in Cluster A [7]. That the co-occurrence of PDs depends critically on the nature of the sample is illustrated by the fact that the co-occurrence of antisocial and borderline PDs varies between 0.3 and 4.0% in the UK and US general population, respectively, but can reach a prevalence of 60% or higher in high-risk criminal samples such as those with 'dangerous and severe personality disorder' (see, e.g., Figure 2.2 in [22]).

Demographic and Psychosocial Correlates

If the prevalence rates of ASPD show some variation, data on the demographic and psychosocial correlates produce a more consistent picture, indicating that the following conclusions may be drawn. First, as we saw earlier, those with ASPD are more likely to be male than female. Second, those with ASPD are generally younger in the population. Third, those with ASPD are more likely to live in an urban environment. Fourth, those with ASPD are likely to be educationally disadvantaged. Fifth, those with ASPD are more likely to be unemployed or have a low income. A single epidemiological investigation which examined the prevalence of ASPD within different ethnic groups found that Native Americans had a prevalence of 11.9%; Blacks, 5.3%; Hispanics, 4.0%; whites, 4.3%; and Asia Pacific Islanders, 1.9% [8]. In the main, ASPD is primarily a disorder of white males. In an 'umbrella review' of risk factors for interpersonal violence in general population samples, it was reported that within the category of personality disorders, ASPD had the strongest link to violence (substance misuse ranked highest among risk factors) [23].

Mortality, Suicide and Suicide Attempts

For the sake of brevity we will consider ASPD and psychopathy together and discuss some interesting comparisons between them. We consider first ASPD and mortality. Three studies have shown that mortality is increased in those with ASPD compared with the general population. First, data from the Epidemiological Catchment Area (ECA) study showed that ASPD was a strong predictor of both mortality from all causes (hazard ratio [HR] = 4.46) and from specific causes, including suicide, chronic lower respiratory disease, and HIV (8.07) [24]. Second, compared with the male Finnish population in general, male criminal offenders with ASPD who were aged under 50 showed a 5- to 9-fold increased risk in general mortality together with a 6- to 17-fold increase in unnatural death (i.e., from suicide, homicide or accident) [25]. Third, a study carried out in in the American state of Iowa followed up 71 men with ASPD over 6–47 years [26]. When compared with age- and gender-matched controls from the general population, ASPD was associated with a particularly high risk of dying. This increased risk persisted throughout all age groups. In summary, there is compelling evidence from these three and other studies that ASPD is associated with increased mortality and that this is especially the case in younger individuals.

In a brief review [27] Martens argued that suicide was such a central feature of ASPD that it ought to be included as one of its diagnostic criteria. However, this is debatable since while, as we saw above, the incidence of suicide is elevated among those with ASPD, it is significantly lower than in other psychiatric disorders [28]. There is compelling evidence, on the other hand, that attempted suicide is common among those with ASPD [28]. Insofar as suicide attempts are positively associated with completed suicides, this unfortunate outcome is an important factor to consider when evaluating an individual with ASPD.

Turning now to psychopathy, although there are fewer studies, there is evidence for increased mortality in psychopathic individuals. A Finnish study [29] compared the mortality of 100 psychopathic individuals (>25 on the PCL-R) with (1) 178 offenders with a PCL-R score of less than 25 and (2) a sample from the general population with a follow-up of 20–30 years. Mortality among the psychopaths was increased fivefold compared with the general population and the cause of death was more violent as compared with the non-psychopathic criminal control group.

As regards suicide and psychopathy, while Cleckley [30] maintained that psychopaths were unlikely to engage in suicidal behaviour (but they frequently made threats of suicide that were rarely carried out), empirical investigations have not confirmed this belief. The few studies that have investigated suicidal behaviour solely among psychopaths have shown that suicidal history is more associated with PCL-R Factor-2 (antisocial deviance) than with Factor-1 (interpersonal/affective). A study examined 313 prison inmates assessed with the PCL-R, DSM and Tellegran's Multidimensional Personality Inventory (MPI) in relation to their previous history of suicide [31]. It found that a history of suicide was associated with PCL-R Factor 2 (but not Factor 1) and with ASPD. MPI negative emotionality and low constraint were associated with both suicidality and antisocial deviance, suggesting that emotional impulsiveness is a vulnerability that is common to both. A subsequent investigation examined whether negative emotionality and low constraint (together with substance misuse) among 682 offenders mediated the relationship between ASPD/ psychopathy and suicidal behaviour [32]. Results indicated that ASPD and the impulsive lifestyle facet of PCL-R were weakly predictive of suicidal behaviour; high negative emotionality and low constraint (but not substance misuse) mediated this relationship. The impulsive/lifestyle features retained an independent predictive effect.

In summary, on the key indices of mortality and suicidality, both ASPD and psychopathy had a positive association, indicating again that these disorders are worthy of mental health professionals' interest. Results indicate that emotional impulsiveness (the conjunction of impulsivity and negative affect) is the likely mechanism through which both ASPD and psychopathy are associated with suicidality. We should note that while emotional impulsiveness is characteristic of PCL-R Factor 2 psychopathy, it is *not* characteristic of Cleckleyan psychopaths, who tend to be bold and emotionally stable (see Chapter 4). Thus while Cleckleyan psychopaths frequently threaten suicide but rarely act on their threats, these are likely used as a means to emotionally manipulate others.

Psychosocial Impairment

Psychosocial impairment arising from the presence of PD was investigated in four of the studies. We focus here on its association with ASPD. Using the World Health Organisation Health and Disability Scale (WHO-DAS-11 [33]), Lenzenweger and colleagues reported that PD was significantly associated with psychosocial impairment, especially with social role impairment (OR = 5.6 for ASPD and 8.5 for borderline PD)

[16]. However, once Axis I comorbidity was controlled, these associations diminished to 1.4 and 1.6, respectively. Trull and colleagues investigated quality of life in their series using the Short Form 12 Health Survey [34], finding that those diagnosed with PD were more likely to show impaired functioning [11]. Coid and colleagues noted that individuals with a Cluster B PD were more likely to have been in local authority or institutional care, to have had a criminal conviction and to have spent time in prison [7].

Results of two other studies that investigated the NESARC-III sample indicated a strong association between substance use and contact with the criminal justice system in US adults [35, 36]. In this same sample, past-year contact with the criminal justice system was present in 10% of those showing antisocial/borderline PD comorbidity but in less than 6% of those showing ASPD alone and less than 1% of those receiving neither an ASPD nor a borderline PD diagnosis [17]. Since both ASPD and borderline PD are highly associated with substance misuse [37], it seems likely that the high level of contact with the criminal justice system in those with both ASPD and borderline PD is due largely to their drug and alcohol misuse. This has implications for efforts aimed at rehabilitating these individuals, suggesting that these efforts should primarily be targeted at reducing their substance misuse.

Service Use

Three of the eight studies selected reported on service use either by cluster or specifically by ASPD. Coid and colleagues' study reported service use by cluster only [7]. They found that although PDs were associated with high service use across a range of health services, these associations disappeared after adjusting for demographics and comorbid Axis I conditions. Like others, they make the point that the high use of services by some in the Cluster B group is due to their comorbid mental illnesses rather than difficulties arising from their PD. Lenzenweger and colleagues' study [16] provides the most detailed information, particularly as they report on service usage by ASPD and borderline PD separately. They found that while 39% of those with any PD reported having treatment over the previous 12 months, this increased to 49.1% for those with a Cluster B disorder. They found, first, that 46.1% of those with ASPD had sought treatment in the previous 12 months; second, that those with ASPD were about five times more likely to have sought treatment compared with those without PD; and, third, that when the effects of comorbid Axis I disorders were controlled, those with PD were less than two times more likely to have sought treatment. They concluded that the increase in treatment seeking of those with ASPD was accounted for to a greater extent by their comorbid mental illness syndromes than by their PD. Finally, Goldstein and colleagues reported on the treatment-seeking behaviour of those with ASPD [8]. Treatment-seeking behaviour was reported to be uncommon in those with ASPD: only 25% sought help with their disorder. Overall, this suggests that, consistent with our previously articulated psychological perspective of this 'disorder', individuals diagnosed with ASPD attribute the source of their difficulties to external rather than internal factors. That is, they blame others rather than themselves for their problematic life trajectory.

Cross-Cultural Variation in ASPD

It has been argued that while the prevalence of all mental disorders varies across cultures, culture is likely to have a greater impact on the prevalence of personality disorders compared with syndromal mental illnesses [38]. While the evidence for this is sparse, it is partly borne out by data, the most reliable evidence coming from studies of antisocial personality disorder [39]. Compton and colleagues reported lifetime prevalence rates of ASPD in Taiwan and the United States using a comparable methodology taken from the Epidemiological Catchment Area Study [40]. They found rates of 0.2% in Taiwan compared with 3% in the United States. Although the same sampling and instrumentation were used in both countries, it is unclear whether the difference in rates was due to method variance, true variance or a combination of both.

Despite the dearth of relevant cross-cultural data that we can draw on, it is clear that the prevalence of ASPD reported in US studies is considerably higher than that reported for European studies. We will see below that this is also true of the prevalence rates of psychopathy. Moreover, rates of ASPD appear to be doubling since World War II [41]. Various hypotheses have been proposed for this increased prevalence of ASPD in the United States. It has been attributed to an increase in substance misuse and family breakdown, and perhaps most importantly, the culture of individualism prevalent in American society, contrasted with the culture of collectivism found in Asian countries [42]. More systematic empirical studies will be required to confirm these hypotheses. Mulder has provided a useful summary of the evidence on cross-cultural differences in ASPD [42]. His conclusions were, first, that ASPD appears to occur ubiquitously across most cultures, albeit at different rates; second, that ASPD is more common in Western cultures; and third, that rates of ASPD, and possibly other PDs, are increasing, with social and cultural factors playing a significant role in this increase.

Summary of Findings from Recent Studies

Recent epidemiological studies reviewed above confirm, albeit in slightly reduced form, earlier prevalence rates of ASPD found in the community. They suggest that individuals with ASPD are predominantly white single young men living in urban environments. They are sociodemographically disadvantaged with multiple comorbid conditions, especially substance misuse. In the unlikely event of seeking treatment, they will do so only for a comorbid condition rather than to address their personality difficulties. Given the grave consequences of the individual's behaviour for himself, for his social network and for the wider community and his reluctance to seek any help, ASPD represents a major challenge to health service provision.

ASPD in Prison Populations

Given that the DSM criteria for ASPD conflate criminal offending (grounds for arrest) with personality variables, it is hardly surprising that ASPD is so prevalent in prison populations. We saw in Chapter 1 that while early studies suggested as many as three-quarters of North American prison inmates qualified for an ASPD diagnosis, more recent data indicate that less than half may do so. Figures for the UK prison population were provided by a survey conducted in 1999 [43]. Personality disorders were diagnosed with SCID-II (DSM-IV) using clinical interviewers. Separate prevalence estimates were provided on sentenced, remanded and women prisoners which were weighted accordingly. Of 3,568 prisoners selected to participate in the research, 88% agreed to be interviewed in an initial screening phase and 76% agreed to undergo a subsequent clinical interview. The prevalence of any PD was 78% for men on remand, 64% for sentenced men, and 50% for women. Prisoners with any PD were more likely to be young, unmarried, of white ethnic origin and to be charged with acquisitive rather than drug offences. ASPD was the most prevalent PD, occurring in 63% of remanded men, 49% of sentenced men and 31% of women. The second most prevalent PD, paranoid PD, occurred in 29% of remanded men, 20% of sentenced men and 16% of women. High rates of comorbidity were found in prisoners generally. Prisoners with ASPD were less likely to suffer from a functional psychosis, but were more likely to report hazardous drinking in the year before imprisonment and were six times more likely to report drug dependence. Those with ASPD were also more likely to be given disciplinary sanctions within the prison. Those with ASPD did not perceive a lack of social support as being a vulnerability factor, suggesting that depending on one's own resources might have been important for prisoners with ASPD.

A broader view of PD, and ASPD in particular, among incarcerated populations was provided by a systematic review of prisoners' mental health in Western countries [44]. These authors reviewed 62 studies from 12 Western countries in which 22,790 prisoners were evaluated. A high prevalence of any PD, and of ASPD in particular, was found among male prisoners: 65% and 47%, respectively. For women, the rates were 42% for any PD and 21% for ASPD. The authors concluded that prisoners were 10 times more likely than the general population to have ASPD.

In summary, while neither necessary nor sufficient for an ASPD diagnosis, criminal behaviour is so integral to its diagnosis that it is no surprise that it is met by roughly one half of prisoners. Considering the high degree of psychosocial impairment and comorbidity found in community studies of ASPD, together with the lack of resources within the custodial system, it is likely that there is a considerable amount of unmet need for mental health intervention within the prison population.

Psychopathy in Prison Populations

As indicated in Chapter 1, roughly a quarter of North American prison inmates qualify for a designation as 'psychopathic' according to a cut score of 30 on the Psychopathy Checklist – Revised (PCL-R). In one of the first transcultural studies comparing Scottish and North American prisoners, Cooke and Michie reported a higher prevalence of psychopathy in the North American than in the Scottish sample [45]. The authors considered various explanations to account for this difference, including cultural differences and different patterns of migration. It was concluded that psychopathy measured by the PCL-R could be validly applied to populations outside North America, albeit with a lower threshold for 'caseness'.

Using a cross-sectional sample taken from the sample in [43] and a PCL-R cut score of 30, Coid and colleagues estimated the prevalence of psychopathy among a representative group of 496 prisoners in the United Kingdom [46]. The prevalence of psychopathy was found to be 7.7% for men and 1.9% for women. Rates were higher among male prisoners on remand (9.4%) compared with sentenced prisoners (6.2%), but this association disappeared after controlling for other demographic factors. Among DSM-IV Axis II disorders, ASPD correlated highly with PCL-R and with all four of its facets. They found significant associations of PCL-R psychopathy with alcohol and drug misuse together with receiving additional punishments because of misbehaviour. They concluded that 'psychopathy identifies the extreme of a spectrum of social and behavioural problems among prisoners' [46, p. 134].

Studies reviewed by Fanti and colleagues consistently showed higher PCL-R psychopathy scores in North American adult prisoners and youth offenders compared with their European (mostly British) counterparts [47]. The effect sizes for these differences were quite substantial, ranging from 0.30 to 0.57 in youth offenders. In attempting to explain these differences, the authors suggested they might be due to a greater tendency in Europe (and in the United Kingdom and Germany in particular) for mentally disordered (especially psychopathic) offenders to be diverted away from the prison system into secure psychiatric facilities. These types of offender, they argue, would more likely end up in prison in North America. However, this explanation would be more plausible if community surveys, considered below, also found a difference between North America and the United Kingdom.

Psychopathy in the Community

There is a dearth of studies that have attempted to assess psychopathy in community samples, which is unfortunate given Cleckley's seminal description of the psychopathic individual as one who survives and prospers in the community [30]. Of 39 studies reviewed by Fanti and colleagues [47] that used the PCL-R or its abbreviated, screening version (the PCL:SV), across 15 countries, only two investigated community samples. Examination of psychopathy in the community has hitherto been limited to several small-scale studies on the distribution of psychopathic traits using self-report measures with opportunistic samples (e.g., university students) or by advertising for paid volunteers who were likely to have the relevant traits [47].

Exceptionally, two community studies using the PCL-R:SV have provided worthwhile data. The first examined a stratified community sample from the MacArthur Violence Risk Assessment Study [48]. Using a cut score of at least 13 on the PLC:SV, these authors reported a prevalence rate of 1.2% for the total sample (1% males, 1.2% females, 1.9% African American and 1% white). The majority had few if any psychopathic traits. PCL:SV psychopathy was found to predict violence, alcohol use and a lower estimated intelligence. The second study [49] examined PCL:SV scores in 638 individuals from the UK Household Survey. The authors reported a weighted prevalence of 0.6% for psychopathy in the population using a cut score of 13 on the PCL:SV. Being younger, male, misusing drugs (but not alcohol) and violent behaviour all correlated positively with the PCL:SV score. As in the first study, psychopathic traits were not normally distributed. Therefore, while the majority did not demonstrate any psychopathic traits, these were evident in a small subgroup.

The difference in the prevalence of psychopathy in the United Kingdom (0.6%) compared with in the United States (>1) corroborates cross-national differences found with ASPD. Notwithstanding these differences, the extant studies in community samples indicate a much lower prevalence of psychopathy among community residents compared with those who have been convicted of an offence and imprisoned. This is not too surprising when one considers that the PCL-R, the standard measure of psychopathy, and ASPD both, in their operational criteria, conflate criminal behaviour with personality deviation. There has been a recent debate concerning whether criminal behaviour is an intrinsic aspect of psychopathy or is a downstream result of psychopathy (e.g., [50]). Evidence discussed in Chapter 1 suggests that contact with the criminal justice system, at least in the United States, exerts a disproportionate influence on an ASPD diagnosis [51]. Of the community sample in this study, 53% had no contact with the criminal justice system, and amongst these the prevalence of ASPD was less than 1%. There seems little doubt that, *as operationally defined* (by a high PCL-R score or by the ASPD criteria), both PCL-R psychopathy and ASPD reflect in no small degree criminality and contact with the criminal justice system. This need not imply that ASPD and psychopathy are synonymous with criminality or equivalent to it. But it does mean that it is imperative to disaggregate criminality from both ASPD and psychopathy if these constructs are to have import as personality constructs, rather than simply re-describing a criminal propensity.

Summary and Conclusions

By examining several more recent and well-conducted community and prison studies, this chapter aimed to update findings on the epidemiology of ASPD since Moran's review appeared some 20 years ago. These more recent findings largely mirror those found in earlier publications. These studies suggest that the prevalence of ASPD in the community is probably less than previously thought, with a prevalence rate of 0.6–1%, although the United States may be an outlier. Those with ASPD also feature prominently among the prison population (around 50%). Our focus has been on community rather than prison samples, emphasising the psychological structure of the disorder rather than the criminality that we regard as an epiphenomenon. The scarce data on the prevalence of psychopathy in the community indicate that it is less prevalent than ASPD, but again the rates are lower in the United Kingdom compared with the United States. Psychopathy is substantially less prevalent in the community than in prison, where its prevalence is around 15–25%.

What lessons can we learn from these epidemiological studies? We suggest the following:

1. ASPD and psychopathy are much more prevalent among criminal than among community samples. As we have indicated, both constructs, ASPD and psychopathy, are conflated with criminality and need to be stripped of their association with criminal behaviour if they are to be meaningful psychological constructs.

2. ASPD is strongly associated with being young, male and socially disadvantaged. Men so diagnosed bear several disadvantages, including being poorly educated, having a low income and being single. They also suffer from multiple comorbidities, most significant among which are alcohol and drug misuse. We suggest it is their drug and alcohol misuse that is largely responsible for these individuals falling into the net of the criminal justice system and particularly for their engaging in violent behaviour. The link between drug and alcohol misuse and antisocial personality is explored further in Chapter 3.

3. Few of these disadvantaged young men seek any treatment, and when they do, it is largely because of co-occurring psychiatric disorders. In the language of Tyrer and colleagues [52], they are treatment rejecting rather than treatment seeking. They therefore represent a significant challenge to anyone who seeks to intervene to alter their life's trajectory. We explore approaches to intervening with these individuals in the following two chapters.

References

1. L. N. Robins, J. T Tipp, T. Prezbeck. Antisocial personality. In: L. N. Robins, D. E. Regier, eds., *Psychiatric Disorders in America*. New York: Free Press, 1991; 258–290.

2. P. Moran. *Antisocial Personality Disorder: An Epidemiological Perspective*. London: Gaskell Press, 1999.

3. J. W. Coid. The diagnostic dilemma: DSM-III diagnosis in criminal psychopaths: A way forward. *Criminal Behaviour and Mental Health* 1992; **2**: 78–94.

4. S. Torgersen, E. Kringlen, V. Cramer. The prevalence of personality disorder in a community sample. *Archives of General Psychiatry* 2001; **58**: 590–596.

5. S. Torgersen. Epidemiology. In: T. A. Widiger, ed., *The Oxford Handbook of Personality Disorders*. New York: Oxford University Press, 2012.

6. B. F. Grant, F. S. Stinson, D. A. Dawson, P. Chou, M. A. Ruan, P. Roger, M. S. Pickering. Co-occurrence of 12-month alcohol and drug use disorders and personality disorders in the United States: Results from the national epidemiologic survey on alcohol and related conditions. *Archives of General Psychiatry* 2004; **61**: 361–368.

7. J. W. Coid, M. Yang, P. Tyrer, A. Roberts, S. Ullrich. Prevalence and correlates of personality disorder in Great Britain. *British Journal of Psychiatry* 2006; **188**: 423–431.

8. R. B Goldstein, P. Chou, T. D. Saha, S. M. Smith, J. Jeesun Jung, H. Zhang, R. P. Pickering, W. J. Ruan, B. J. Huang. B. F. Grant. The epidemiology of antisocial behavioral syndromes in adulthood: Results from the National Epidemiologic Survey on Alcohol and Related Conditions. *Journal of Clinical Psychiatry* 2017; **78**: 90–98.

9. A. W. Loranger, N. Sartorius, A. Andreoli, P. Berger, P. Buchheim, S. M. Channabasavanna, et al. The International Personality Disorder Examination (IPDE). The World Health Organization/Alcohol, Drug Abuse, and Mental Health Administration international pilot study of personality disorders. *Archives of General Psychiatry* 1994; **51**: 21.

10. J. Samuals, W. W. Eaton, O. J. Bienvenu, C. H. Brown, P. T. Costa, G. Nestadt. Prevalence and correlates of personality disorders in a community sample. *British Journal of Psychiatry* 2002; **188**: 536–542.

11. T. J. Trull, S. Jahng, R. L. Tomko, P. K. Wood, K. J. Sher. Revised NESARC personality disorder diagnoses: Gender, prevalence, and comorbidity with substance dependence disorders. *Journal of Personality Disorders* 2010; **24**: 412–426.

12. L. N. Robins, D. A. Regier. *Psychiatric Disorders in America*. New York: Free Press, 1991.

13. B. Bishop, B. Völlm, N. Khalifa. Women with antisocial personality disorder. In: D. W. Black, N. Kolla, eds., *Textbook of Antisocial Personality Disorder*. Washington, DC: American Psychiatric Press, 2021.

14. O. V. Berkout, J. N. Young, A. M. Gross. Mean girls and bad boys: Recent research on gender differences in conduct disorder. *Aggression and Violent Behavior* 2011; **16**: 503–511. https://doi.org/10.1016/j.avb.2011.06.001.

15. A. A. Alegria, C. Blanco, N. M. Petry, A. E. Skodol, S. M. Liu, B. Grant. Sex differences in antisocial personality disorder: Results from the national epidemiological study on alcohol and related conditions. *Personality Disorders: Theory, Research, and Treatment* 2013; **4**: 214–222. doi: 10.1037/a0031681.

16. M. F Lenzenweger, M. C. Lane, A. W. Loranger, R. C. Kessler. DSM-IV personality disorders in the National Comorbidity Survey Replication. *Biological Psychiatry* 2007; **62**: 553–564.

17. R. C. Howard, D. Hasin, M. Stohl. Substance use disorders and criminal justice contact among those with co-occurring antisocial and borderline personality disorders: Findings from a

nationally representative sample. *Personality and Mental Health* 2020. https://doi.org/10.1002/pmh.1491.

18. T. A. Widiger, T. J. Trull. Plate tectonics in the classification of personality disorder: Shifting to a dimensional model. *American Psychologist* 2007; **62**: 71–83.

19. S. O. Lilienfeld, I. D. Waldman, A. C. Israel. A critical examination of the use of the term and concept of *comorbidity* in psychopathology research. *Clinical Psychology: Science and Practice* 1994; 1: 71–83.

20. W. J. Livesley. Conceptual issues. In: W. J. Livesley, R. Larstone, eds., *Handbook of Personality Disorders*, 2nd ed. New York: Guilford Press, 2018; 3–24.

21. T. J. Trull, E. M. Scheiderer, R. L. Tomko. Axis II comorbidity. In: T. A. Widiger, ed., *The Oxford Handbook of Personality Disorders*. New York: Oxford University Press, 2012; 219–236.

22. C. Duggan, R. Howard. The 'functional link' between personality disorder and violence. In M. McMurran, R. C. Howard, eds., *Personality, Personality Disorder and Violence*. Chichester: John Wiley & Sons, 2009; 19–37.

23. S. Fazel, N. Smith, C. Cheng, J. Geddes, Risk factors for interpersonal violence: An umbrella review of meta-analyses. *British Journal of Psychiatry* 2018; **213**: 609–614.

24. A. Krasnova, W. W. Eaton, J. F. Samuels. Antisocial personality and risks of cause-specific mortality: Results from the Epidemiologic Catchment Area study with 27 years of follow up. *Social Psychiatry and Psychiatric Epidemiology* 2019; **54**: 617–625.

25. E. Repo-Tiihonen, M. Virkkunen, J. Tiihonen. Mortality of antisocial male criminals. *The Journal of Forensic Psychiatry* 2001; **12**: 677–683.

26. D. W. Black, C. H. Baumgard, S. E. Bell. Death rates in 71 men with antisocial personality disorder: A comparison with general population mortality. *Psychosomatics* 1996; **37**: 131–136.

27. W. H. J. Martens. Suicidal behaviour as an essential diagnostic feature of antisocial personality disorder. *Psychopathology* 2001; **34**: 274–275.

28. M. J. Garvey, F. Spoden. Suicide attempts in antisocial personality disorder. *Comprehensive Psychiatry* 1980; **21**: 146–149.

29. O. Vaurio, E. Repo-Tiihonen, H. Kautiainen, J. Tiihonen. Psychopathy and mortality. *Journal of Forensic Science* 2018; **63**: 474–477.

30. H. Cleckley. *The Mask of Sanity*, 5th ed. St Louis, MO: Mosby, 1976 (originally published in 1941).

31. E. Verona, C. J. Patrick, T. E. Joiner. Psychopathy, antisocial personality, and suicide risk. *Journal of Abnormal Psychology* 2001; **110**: 462–470.

32. K. S. Douglas, J. L. Skeem, N. G. Poythress, J. F. Edens, C. J. Patrick. Relation of antisocial and psychopathic traits to suicide-related behavior among offenders. *Law and Human Behavior* 2008; **32**: 511–525.

33. L. A. Chwastiak, M. Von Korf. Disability in depression and back pain: Evaluation of the World Health Organization Disability Assessment Schedule (WHO DAS II) in a primary care setting. *Journal of Clinical Epidemiology* 2003; **56**: 507–514.

34. J. E. Ware, M. Kosinkski, D. M. Turner-Bowker, B. Gandek. *How to Score Version 2 of the SF-12 Health Survey*. Lincoln, RI: Quality Metrics, 2002.

35. K. E. Moore, L. M. S. Oberleitner, H. V. Zonana, A. W. Buchanan, B. P. Pittman, T. L. Verplaetse, et al. Psychiatric disorders and crime in the US population: Results from the National Epidemiologic Survey on Alcohol and Related Conditions Wave III. *Journal of Clinical Psychiatry* 2019; **28**: 165–172. https://doi.org/10.4088/JCP.18m12317.

36. K. E. Moore, L. M. S. Oberleitner, B. P. Pittman, W. Roberts, T. L. Verplaetse, R. L. Hacker, et al. The prevalence of substance use disorders among community-based adults with legal

problems in the U.S. *Addiction Research & Theory* 2019; **28**: 165–172. https://doi.org/10.1080/16066359.2019.1613524.

37. P. Köck, M. Walter. Personality disorder and substance use disorder: An update. *Mental Health & Prevention* 2018; **12**: 82–89.

38. J. G. Draguns. Culture and psychopathology: What is known about their relationship? *Australian Journal of Psychology* 1986; **38**: 329–338.

39. J. Paris. Personality disorders in sociocultural perspective. *Journal of Personality Disorders* 1998; **12**: 289–301.

40. W. M. Compton, J. E. Helzer, H. G. Hwu, E. K. Yeh, L. McEvoy, J. E. Tipp, E. L. Spitznagal. New methods in cross-cultural psychiatry: Psychiatric illness in Taiwan and the United States. *American Journal of Psychiatry* 1991; **148**: 1697–1704.

41. R. C. Kessler, K. A. McGonagle, S. Zhao, C. B. Nelson, M. Hughes, S. Eshleman, K. S. Kendler. Lifetime and 12-month prevalence of DSM-III-R psychiatric disorders in the United States. Results from the National Comorbidity Survey. *Archives of General Psychiatry* 1994; **51**: 8–19.

42. R. T. Mulder. Cultural aspects of personality disorder. In T. A. Widiger, ed., *The Oxford Handbook of Personality Disorders*. New York: Oxford University Press, 2012; 260–274.

43. N. Singleton, H. Meltze, R. Gatward, J. Coid, D. Deasy. *Psychiatric Morbidity among Prisoners in England and Wales*. London: The Stationery Office, 1998.

44. S. Fazel, J. Danesh. Serious mental disorder in 23000 prisoners: A systematic review of 62 surveys. *The Lancet* 2019; **359**: 545–550.

45. D. J. Cooke, C. Michie. Psychopathy across cultures: North America and Scotland compared. *Journal of Abnormal Psychology* 1999; **108**: 58–68.

46. J. Coid et al. Psychopathy among prisoners in England and Wales. *International Journal of Law and Psychiatry* 32: 134–141.

47. K. A. Fanti, A. Lordos, E. A. Sullivan, D. S. Kosson. Cultural and ethnic variations in psychopathy. In: C. J. Patrick, ed., *Handbook of Psychopathy*, 2nd ed. New York: Guilford Press, 2018; 529–569.

48. C. S. Neumann, R. D. Hare. Psychopathic traits in a large community sample: Links to violence, alcohol use and intelligence. *Journal of Consulting and Clinical Psychology* 2008; 76, 5: 893–899.

49. J. Coid, M. Yang, S. Ullrich, A. Roberts, R. D. Hare. Prevalence and correlates of psychopathic traits in the household population of Great Britain. *International Journal of Law and Psychiatry* 2009; 32, 2: 65–73.

50. D. J. Cooke. Psychopathic personality in different cultures: What do we know? What do we need to find out? *Journal of Personality Disorders* 1996; **10**: 23–40.

51. J. Schnittker, S. H. Larimore, H. Lee. Neither mad nor bad? The classification of antisocial personality disorder among formerly incarcerated adults. *Social Science & Medicine*; 2020. doi: 10.1016/j.socscimed.2020.113288.

52. P. Tyrer, S. Mitchard, C. Methuen, M. Ranger. Treatment rejecting and treatment seeking personality disorders: Type R and type S. *Journal of Personality Disorders* 2003; **17**: 263–268.

Treatment of ASPD, Part 1
General Approaches

Overview

This chapter focuses on the principles and practices of treating those with ASPD from the perspective of (1) a generalist (i.e., professionals or service providers who lack specialist skills or training) and (2) obtaining engagement and providing emotional stability to the participant. It first reviews the evidence from two Cochrane Systematic Reviews for the effectiveness of psychological and pharmacological interventions for those with ASPD.

As the evidence for specific interventions from good quality trials is weak, we propose a pragmatic alternative that relies on (1) the non-specific effects of psychotherapy and (2) the construction of a case conceptualisation that guides whichever interventions are offered. The non-specific factors in psychotherapy encompass a triad of (1) establishing and maintaining a therapeutic relationship, (2) the creation of expectations through an explanation of the disorder and (3) the enactment of health-promoting actions – each of which is considered in detail together with the supplemental use of medications. A case conceptualisation (or clinical formulation) is then expanded into its component parts. We believe that this phased approach allows practitioners, who often have limited resources, to manage those with ASPD in a sensible and defensible manner. Both the non-specific effects of psychotherapy and the case conceptualization are influenced by the 'tripartite self' discussed in previous chapters.

Introduction

Treating someone with ASPD automatically raises the question, What is the objective of the intervention? Is it a significant refashioning of the individual's personality such that whatever dysfunction caused by the pathological personality traits is reduced? Or is it a more modest aim of dampening down the consequences of the more extreme behaviours while leaving the core personality unchanged? One must also recognise that ASPD represents a spectrum of severity with some presenting with mild but persistent anti-social behaviours while others portray a more severe disorder. It is likely therefore that several different approaches may be necessary to deal with problems across this range of severity.

In addition, the answer to the question of 'What is the objective of the intervention?' is very much dependent on the interests of the questioner. For instance, a forensic psychologist might be satisfied if further recidivism was reduced by treatment, whereas an abused spouse might wish to have a reduction in physical aggression and, perhaps, even some intimacy in the relationship. The issue of co-morbidity also comes into play in that successful control of excessive alcohol or drug misuse is likely to have a secondary positive effect in reducing violence and acquisitive offending. Finally, there is the issue of allocation of resources. Should one, for instance, concentrate one's resources on a relatively small number of serious cases, providing them with extensive and costly interventions even if this is at the expense of providing simpler and less costly interventions for a much larger group that may be less severely affected?

In summary, recommending interventions for ASPD and assessing their efficacy is complex and can be approached at a number of levels. This (and the subsequent chapter) will attempt to tease out these issues and provide some practical guidance in managing this challenging population.

In addition to the dilemmas described above, there is the question of how to assess the evidence of efficacy when making recommendations for treatment. For instance, it is now commonly accepted that one should adopt an 'evidence-based' approach in the choice of intervention. This should ideally depend on information from a number of systematic reviews and meta-analyses, exemplified by the Cochrane Systematic Review and NICE Guidelines, that rigorously assess the best available evidence against pre-defined criteria to produce treatment guidelines. Two such Cochrane reviews have been published on ASPD, one on psychological [1] and the other on pharmacological [2] interventions. While both rigorous and helpful in scoping the evidence available, these reviews are of limited practical value to the practitioner since the trials considered were, in the view of the reviewers, few in number and methodologically flawed. Nonetheless, this evidence base will be briefly considered in this chapter as it at least provides a benchmark for the conduct of future investigations.

While the absence of clear evidence on which to base one's recommendations for treating ASPD is problematic, it is not unique to that condition. The alternative then is to develop a sensible approach which incorporates what we know conceptually and empirically about ASPD to produce a workable treatment plan. Given the absence of good-quality trial evidence, this approach is not ideal but does at least have the following advantages. First, it departs from an overtly medicalised conceptualisation of PD which has been criticised as not being appropriate for personality disorder [3]. Second, it is recognised even by advocates of an evidence-based approach that the evidence needs to be tempered for each individual case. For instance, Sackett et al. define evidence-based medicine as 'the conscientious, explicit, and judicious use of *current best evidence* in making decisions *about the care of individual patients*' (emphasis added) thereby taking account of the individuality of the patient when applying it [4]. Relevant here are McAdams' [5] concepts of 'self as autobiographical author' and 'self as motivated agent' referred to in Chapters 1 and 2 (see Figure 2.2), and expanded on in the final chapter. In such cases, it may be important to look beyond signs and symptoms, and instead probe the person's biographical narrative [6, 7]. While Sackett and colleagues emphasise the importance of using 'individual clinical expertise' to apply this external evidence to an individual case, there is little written about how this might actually be done in practice; this aspect will be addressed in this chapter.

The third advantage of an alternative eclectic approach is that it allows practitioners who might have a particular interest in a specific intervention to adopt whichever modality of treatment best accords with their therapeutic interest. This has the advantage of personal commitment on the part of the practitioner, which as we will see in the following chapter counts for a great deal in the eventual outcome. This eclectic approach, however, is open to the criticism that it allows practitioners to adopt whichever treatment takes their fancy without good evidence to support it, a situation that is clearly unsatisfactory.

Producing evidence for the practitioner therefore needs to strike a balance between, on the one hand, a reliance on whatever scanty scientific evidence exists and, on the other hand, producing sensible guidance that is both rational and defensible. We will first review the evidence from the Cochrane Systematic Reviews before proceeding to outline an approach which can be applied by practitioners in non-specialist settings. In the chapter that follows we will consider more specialist interventions that focus on the management of violence and criminality, particularly in secure settings.

Since our current focus is on adults with ASPD, interventions for children and adolescents, important in preventing the progression from childhood conduct disorder to adult ASPD, will not be considered. This area has been comprehensively covered in the NICE Guidance on ASPD, together with its updates to which the interested reader may refer [8]. Further, since we concur with others (e.g., [3]) that the primary therapy for ASPD is psychological rather than pharmacological, the main focus of this chapter is on psychological treatments, with drug treatments playing at most a supplementary role.

Treatment Efficacy

Psychological Interventions

Evidence for psychological interventions for ASPD was reviewed by Gibbon and colleagues [1] – an update of their previous review[9]. This later review included 19 studies where the selection criterion was random assignment to the psychological intervention against 'treatment as usual' (TAU), also called 'standard maintenance' (SM) in some studies. Their primary outcomes were aggression, reconviction, global state/functioning, social functioning and adverse events. There were only four studies that focussed exclusively on those with ASPD; the remaining 15 focussed on subgroups of participants with ASPD.

Results: A brief summary of the results of this review is as follows.

1. One study examined the effectiveness of cognitive behavioural therapy (CBT) in reducing physical aggression and another on improving social functioning. Neither showed any benefit at 12-month follow-up.
2. Similarly, impulsive lifetime counselling (ILC) + TAU versus TAU alone showed no difference on trait aggression at 9-month follow-up while another (using the same intervention) showed no evidence of benefit on the adverse event of death and 'very low certainty evidence' of a reduction of incarceration between 3 and 9 months of follow-up.
3. One study that examined the benefits of contingency management (CM) + SM versus SM alone on the social functioning of addicts on the Addiction Severity Index showed 'very low certainty evidence' of benefit at 6 months.
4. Again, with a similar group, a 'driving whilst intoxicated' (DWI) programme + incarceration versus incarceration alone showed no difference for prisoner participants on their reconviction rates at 24 months.
5. A study comparing schema therapy (ST) versus TAU found no difference in the reconviction rates or overall adverse events at 3 years, although there was an improvement in social functioning.

6. Another study examined social problem-solving (SPS) + psychoeducation (PE) versus TAU and found no difference in the level of social functioning at 6 months' post intervention.
7. One study using dialectical behavioural therapy with 14 participants with a low certainty indication provided very low-certainty evidence that the intervention reduced the number of self-harm days for outpatients at 2 months' post-intervention compared with TAU.
8. A final small study (with 35 participants) found no evidence of a difference between psychosocial risk management (PSRM; 'Resettlement Programme') and TAU for the number of offences after 1 year after release from prison or in the number of adverse events of death.

In summarising their findings from this review, the authors write as follows: 'The current review concludes that good-quality evidence in favour of any psychological intervention for ASPD continues to be virtually non-existent.'

Pharmacological Interventions

Khalifa and colleagues reported on treatment efficacy of pharmacological agents for ASPD in another Cochrane Systematic Review that considered 11 trials with 416 participants with ASPD; however, data were available from only four studies involving 274 participants [2]. This again was an update of a previous review published in 2010 [10]. Participants in most of the studies presented primarily with substance misuse and no study recruited participants with ASPD alone. None of the studies recruited participants who had ASPD alone. Participants with ASPD were randomly assigned either to a pharmacological agent (e.g., antiepileptic, antidepressant or dopamine agonist [anti-Parkinsonian] drug) or to a placebo control. The outcome variables included aggression, anger, global/state functioning, social functioning and substance misuse (including alcohol dependence); none measured reconviction as an outcome.

Results: One study (60 participants) reported that phenytoin (300 mg/day), compared with placebo, 'may' reduce the mean frequency of aggressive acts per week in prisoners. Neither desipramine nor nortriptyline was effective in improving the social functioning scores among those with alcohol dependency. Bromocriptine (a dopamine agonist) again showed no difference on mean global state functioning scores compared with placebo, but 12 of the 18 patients randomised to the bromocriptine group experienced severe side effects, five of whom dropped out of the study in the first two days due to nausea and severe flu-like symptoms.

None of the findings was replicated and overall the study quality was poor. The authors' conclusion was similar to that of their companion study of psychological treatments in that there was insufficient evidence to recommend the use of pharmacotherapy for those with ASPD.

Summary

Little if any good evidence supported the use of either psychological or pharmacological interventions for ASPD from these two reviews. The trials considered were generally of poor quality, under-powered and focused on associated features of ASPD (i.e., substance misuse) rather than the core characteristics of ASPD.

As regards the pharmacological interventions, it is striking how dated are the drugs which were evaluated. For instance, if one compares the drugs evaluated in the Khalifa review against the recommendations of the Seiver and Davis review discussed below [11], one finds that many of the recommendations (e.g., selective serotonin reuptake inhibitors [SSRIs], more recent anti-convulsants, anti-psychotics) have not been evaluated. We regard this as a serious omission as the unwary may be led to believe that medication has no role in this disorder, whereas, on the basis of the current evidence, we simply do not know.

The psychological treatments suffer to a lesser extent from this criticism as they consider interventions such as DBT, CBT, CT and ST which are commonplace as psychological interventions for many with personality disorder. Nonetheless, the authors acknowledge that this list is incomplete as interventions such as mentalizing-based therapy, therapeutic community treatment, cognitive analytic therapy, and nidotherapy were not considered as there were no trials that satisfied their criteria for inclusion at the time of their review. No doubt, this omission will be addressed in future revisions.

If one puts this omission to one side, there is another which we would wish to highlight. As the epidemiological evidence cited in the previous chapter highlights that those with ASPD suffer from a number of deficits (including early deprivation, abuse, substance misuse, etc.) it would be unlikely that one specific intervention would address these multiple deficits. Hence, what is required is a much wider lens that encompasses this range of deficits that comprise ASPD and which we propose as a sensible provision for this particular population.

Provision for ASPD in Non-Specialised Settings

What follows is premised on much of what has already been described in this book. As we saw in Chapter 5, the epidemiology of ASPD highlights its prevalence among young men with multiple social disadvantages who are unlikely to seek treatment except, perhaps, for a comorbid condition or when inveigled to do so at the behest of a family member or as a condition mandated by the court. It might therefore be argued that government policy aimed at improving the individual's social circumstances might be far more effective than any therapeutic intervention. While this may be true, we would argue that having an insight into what motivates those with ASPD (i.e., its psychological construct) is essential in getting a 'buy-in' to whatever assistance is provided by whichever agency.

The core psychological construct of ASPD has been considered in Chapter 2 with a suggested tripartite structure that comprises (1) antisocial personality traits,, (2) a motivational component (i.e., in the case of someone with ASPD, a reliance on self to achieve one's aims by whatever means necessary) and (3) a narrative which incorporates the unique features of the individual's life (see Figure 2.2). These three components need to be woven together in a case conceptualisation that we shall describe below. Before doing so, we will discuss some of the non-specific effects of psychotherapy as these have a particular resonance for the non-specialist. In the following chapter, we will concentrate on specialist settings where specific effects are more relevant. The distinction between non-specific and specific effects is, of course, somewhat arbitrary in its practical application as the specialist will also rely on non-specific effects while making any intervention in addition to using some specialist techniques. Nonetheless, while the distinction is not watertight, we will use it to structure this discussion. We start by addressing two questions: Why are non-specific effects important in psychological interventions? and What are they?

Non-Specific Effects in Psychotherapy

Non-specific effects in psychotherapy are important as they explain a large proportion of the variance in the outcome of whichever form of psychotherapy is used. For instance, it has been estimated that the success of a psychotherapy outcome can be partitioned as follows: (1) 40% is due to the patient's pathology and the environmental influences that aid their recovery; (2) 30% is due to the non-specific effects of psychotherapy; (3) 15% is due to the patient's expectation of help and their belief in the rationale and effectiveness of the intervention; and (4) 15% is due to specific effects of the psychotherapy [12]. If one accepts this quadripartite division, two important conclusions are apparent. First, the therapist needs to attend actively both to the patient's unique pathology and to the patient's circumstances as these have the greatest influence on outcome. Second, the non-specific effects (and here we include expectancy as a non-specific effect) substantially outweigh the specific effects in their importance as they contribute 45% of the variance in the outcome. This is not to say that the specific effects or technique are unimportant (see below) but rather that, taken in the round, the non-specific effects are those which any non-specialist ought to attend to.

This being the case, the next question is: What are these non-specific effects and how do they mediate the outcome of treatment? There is a considerable literature on this topic (see [13]). We will concentrate on Wempold's 'contextual model', which describes the following three pathways through which the non-specific effects of psychotherapy produce benefits [14]. These encompass (1) establishing a real relationship, (2) the creation of expectations through an explanation of the disorder and the treatment involved and (3) the enactment of health-promoting actions. We will now consider these in turn.

Establishing a Real Relationship in the Initial Encounter: The Challenge of Engagement

The idiom 'First catch your hare', which is thought to have originated in a recipe for hare soup in Mrs Glasse's *Art of Cookery* (1747) [15], aptly describes the challenge of engaging someone with ASPD in the therapeutic process. Put simply, it means making sure that you have caught your hare before you begin to make the soup. In other words, make sure you have engaged the individual in a meaningful relationship before you progress to the next stage. Given the range of vulnerabilities that someone with ASPD might exhibit, this is no mean undertaking and deserves careful consideration. In all individual therapies, there is an initial encounter between therapist and patient. Wempold describes this initial encounter well:

> The initial meeting of patient and therapist is essentially the meeting of two strangers, with the patient making a determination of whether the therapist is trustworthy, has the necessary expertise, and will take the time and effort to understand both the problem and the context in which the patient and the problem are situated. [14, p. 271]

These aspects have a particular resonance for someone with ASPD as they are likely to be distrustful of the therapist's motives while desiring to maintain their hard-won independence. The pragmatic question is: How should the therapist manage this initial encounter? While there are various ways of achieving engagement, one that we have found to be especially useful is to commence by identifying the abnormal personality traits that might underpin the individual's problems (in this case, the traits listed in Figure 2.1). While one way of doing so would be to assess the individual with one of the accepted personality disorder assessment devices (i.e., SCID-II or IPDE), we recognise that most non-specialists will have neither the time nor the inclination to carry out such an assessment. Nonetheless, what is essential is that the assessor is knowledgeable about: (1) the criteria for a diagnosis of ASPD (Box 1.2 in Chapter 1) or dissocial PD and (2) its likely associated PD comorbidities (borderline, narcissistic and paranoid PDs) and comorbid syndromal conditions – especially substance misuse and affective disorder. It is important to be thorough as this is likely to give the patient the sense that one is both serious and knowledgeable about one's task. For those who are unfamiliar with the criteria for the different disorders, these can be downloaded from the web with operational criteria which are useful for the novice as they act as an aide-memoire and give confidence that one is on the right track.

As an aside, we fear that there is no easy way around this since being unfamiliar with the criteria of ASPD, and how they might impact on the individual's life, is equivalent to someone assessing an individual with chest pain and having no knowledge of the symptoms of either respiratory or cardiac conditions. In both cases, it is clear to the individual being assessed that the assessor is floundering. Some may believe that seeking confirmation of an unfavourable list of characteristics is an unlikely way of building a therapeutic relationship. However, our experience is the reverse insofar as – contrary to expectations – an in-depth knowledge and exploration of the meaning of the criteria of ASPD leads to: (1) a respect for the individual with ASPD by the therapist and (2) an exploration of the individual's problems This can lead to a mutual understanding of the individual's difficulties and can therefore act as valuable glue to hold the therapeutic relationship together. After all, the individual is probably the most aware of their abnormal traits and their consequences (although they may wish to blame others for their presence), so that to ignore or downplay their significance is not credible. Thus, rather than seeing the ASPD criteria as boxes to be ticked, it is preferable to see them as providing a canvas to explore the individual's difficulties. It also has the advantage that if there is a disagreement between the parties as to whether a particular trait is or is not salient, then this disagreement can be discussed and hopefully resolved. We accept that we may be criticised for this preference for the DSM-5 criteria of ASPD rather than other conceptualisations. Our response is twofold. First, the approach which we are recommending here is sufficiently flexible to encompass whichever diagnostic system is chosen. Further, we are aware that these criteria are likely to change with further revisions of both DSM and ICD so that any therapeutic approach needs to be sufficiently adaptable to address such revisions. Second, we believe that the practising clinician needs some form of typology which provides an essential scaffold in order to carry out therapeutic work.

Nonetheless, exploring the individual's difficulties in this manner is likely to produce some challenges. The following example is not atypical.

Clinical Vignette: X was convicted of a sexual homicide after he had strangled his ex-girlfriend. He managed to avoid a prison sentence by 'conning' a psychiatrist and his clinical team that he was psychotic and was sent to a high-secure hospital for 'treatment'.

His fabrication was admitted to and he was re-classified as having a personality disorder. He continued to be detained in high-secure care for 30 years, being moved between different hospitals because of illicit relationships with female staff and other patients. Eventually, he was transferred to medium-secure care where, again, his deceit became evident as he continued to develop relationships with vulnerable women. As he could not be trusted and his future risk could not be confidently assessed, he was confined to long-term secure care without the possibility of discharge.

Although this is an extreme case, it does demonstrate two features of the ASPD deception criterion (i.e., repeated lying and conning others for personal profit or pleasure). Given that the trait, from the collateral history if not from the individual directly, is both persistent and pervasive, how does the assessor respond to patients who say they are not habitually untruthful? What clearly should *not* be done, especially if one has to engage therapeutically with an individual over an extended period of time, is to ignore this issue, as to do so would be to disregard an important piece of information. On the other hand, accusing the individual outright of lying is likely to irreparably harm development of the therapeutic relationship. Here, one needs to steer a middle course. So, the therapist might say: 'I have two different sources of information, can you help me to understand the discrepancy?' Hence exploration, rather than confrontation, is the essential modus operandi at this stage. The therapist will also need to keep in mind that someone who habitually lies is unlikely to behave differently with their therapist (see below discussion of 'therapeutic ruptures').

An alternative scenario concerns verifying the history through third-party information. Those who work in a forensic context are at an advantage here as they will usually have file information (in addition to that from other informants) that provides a more comprehensive and verifiable background. Conversely, those who work in less specialised settings are less fortunate as the only informant may be the patient. In the assessment of those with ASPD, this may be an issue as there is evidence that informants may provide more accurate information than the patient [16]. Suppose then that the therapist seeks additional third-party information but that access to this is then denied by the patient. How does the therapist respond? Here, again, it would be unwise to force the issue at this early stage of engagement as this type of confrontation is unlikely to end well. It might be more productive to say: 'This is obviously a sensitive issue for you, so that, for the moment, it may be best to put this issue to one side, but I think that it is important and that it is something that we will need to return to in the future.'

One further caveat needs to be mentioned, namely, that the initial encounter is not set in stone and may need revision as the therapy proceeds. This can occur for two reasons: (1) the therapist is not in tune with the individual and so misses out on some vital information or (2) the individual deliberately or unconsciously conceals some information from the therapist. It is important therefore that both parties see this as an ongoing dialogue where new information is likely to emerge that will need to be integrated into a revised case conceptualisation or formulation. Indeed, as we will see below when we consider therapeutic ruptures, failure to appreciate that one is on the wrong track can have a very detrimental effect on the work. Despite all of these considerations, the aim of the initial encounter is to produce some common and agreed understanding of the individual's difficulties together with some rationale whereby these might be addressed.

Creation of Expectations through Explanation of the Disorder and the Treatment Involved

Once an agreed understanding of the individual's difficulties has been established in (1) above, the next logical step is, first, to explain the occurrence of the disorder in the individual (i.e., its aetiology) and, second, to outline what might be done to alleviate it (i.e., the anticipated interventions). With a patient diagnosed with ASPD, managing an explanation of the disorder is undoubtedly a challenge. For example, there may be a strong family history of antisocial behaviour extending through several generations. Such a familial history might encourage the individual to disclaim any responsibility for their own behaviour. This needs to be confronted since, however disadvantageous the individual's background, it is essential that they take responsibility for their current behaviour. To do otherwise is to support them in a victim role which will do no one any favours. This issue can be addressed by a statement such as:

> 'Looking at your history, it is clear that you have suffered from several disadvantages such as . . . [giving specific details here is helpful in building a therapeutic alliance as it makes it clear that the therapist is in tune with the patient]. Nonetheless, given the difficulties that you are now faced with, what is most important is that you take responsibility for your behaviour so that we can work together to address it.'

This not only establishes agency where it belongs but more importantly indicates that, despite the background difficulties, the therapist has confidence that the individual's problems can be overcome. This conveys optimism that the situation, with considerable effort from both parties, can be remedied.

However, words are simple and need to be followed by a definite programme that will address difficulties that by definition are long-standing. Several factors come into play here, one being the question of why this person is seeking treatment at this particular time. Is it because a family member or the court has mandated that someone gets treated (or else)? While not to be dismissed, these external pressures are likely to have little impact once the sanction is lifted. Hence the therapist needs to broaden the inquiry to include potential benefits of a particular course of action to both the individual and anyone the individual may have hurt. This is less difficult than it might appear: it should be clear from the initial encounter which behaviours need to be addressed immediately in order that risk might be reduced and the individual might achieve some sense of success. For instance, in the case of problems with impetuous behaviour, a problem-solving approach might be appropriate; in the case of substance misuse, referral to an appropriate agency might be warranted; in the case of angry outbursts, referral to an anger management intervention might be appropriate; and so forth.

We emphasise two points here. First, and most important, these interventions are largely skills based and, being non-confrontational, are generally acceptable to the patient. It is essential in this first phase to avoid addressing the core psychopathology directly as this is likely to provoke a negative reaction. The strategy here is not to change the personality directly but rather to mitigate some of the difficulties arising from the personality constellation. This mitigation will provide both immediate relief and positive gains which are essential if one is to progress further. Second, we believe that this provision will have wide applicability, both in most community mental health teams and even in primary care when this is appropriately resourced. Clearly, many of these antisocial individuals will have multiple needs so that some judgement is needed both as to which ought to have immediate priority and having regard to the resources available. What we are proposing then is that the non-specialist (e.g., primary care physician, general psychiatrist, psychologist, nurse practitioner) is equipped with sufficient knowledge first to conduct a proper assessment of someone with ASPD and second to signpost the individual's needs such that these are met with the resources available. As we will see below, adjunctive medication may also play an important role in facilitating engagement. Clearly, at this stage, the emphasis is on gaining emotional stability rather than more significant changes in the personality structure (these are considered in the next chapter). For many, this may be as much as can be achieved given the limited resources available. This tripartite approach of assessment/psychoeducation progressing to a skills-based approach to a more significant re-structuring of the individual's personality is in accord we believe with Livesley's approach [3] (see Figure 6.1). It is also in accord with whatever resources might be available in particular locations.

The Enactment of Health-Promoting Actions

The third pathway in Wempold's contextual model (corresponding to phase 2 in Figure 6.1) concerns specific actions that patients are expected to engage in and that are expected to result in benefits to them. Examples provided include seeing the world from another's perspective (mentalising therapy), identifying and challenging dysfunctional beliefs (cognitive behavioural therapy) and improving social functioning

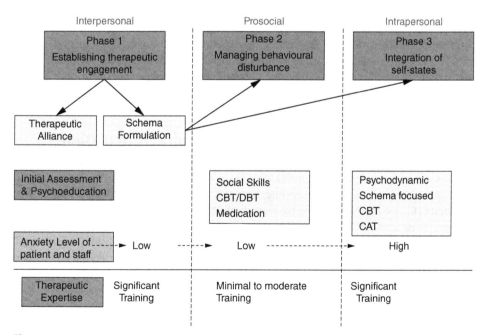

Figure 6.1 A stepped-care approach in the treatment of personality disorder. CAT, cognitive analytic therapy; CBT, cognitive behavioral therapy; DBT, dialectical behavioral therapy.

(interpersonal therapy), in addition of course to ceasing use of illicit substances. These in turn relate to making concrete elements of the treatment approach and in generating hope. According to the contextual model, if these health-promoting actions are undertaken, then benefits are likely to accrue.

Adjunctive Use of Medication

Notwithstanding a lack of supportive evidence [2], the use of medication should not be dismissed out of hand and is more complex than is first apparent for several reasons. First, many patients expect psychiatrists or primary care physicians to prescribe medication if they are in distress. After all, this is what doctors generally do. Clearly, just because these expectations are there does not mean that they should be acceded to. On the contrary, they should be resisted, but not dismissed out of hand. At the very least, the individual ought to be offered an explanation as to why whatever is desired is not being prescribed.

There are two reasons why medication should be considered as an adjunct to treatment. First, evidence firmly supports a common co-occurrence of PD with mental illness and such comorbidity is the rule rather than the exception. When it occurs comorbidly with a PD the mental illness has a worse outcome than in the absence of comorbidity [17]. Hence, it is vital that the therapist carefully assesses whether a mental illness is present. This can easily be missed if the presence of ASPD is salient to such a degree that the mental illness is overlooked. Furthermore, since mental illness is likely to be more challenging to treat in the context of co-occurring PD [17], it may require the continuation of appropriate pharmacotherapy beyond what is suggested in current guidelines. Second, despite the small evidence base for pharmacotherapy in ASPD, Siever and Davis suggest how difficulties in three symptom areas might be treated with medication [11]. These areas are: (1) cognitive perceptual difficulties, (2) impulsive behavioural dyscontrol and (3) affective dysregulation. For instance, for an individual with ASPD and primarily paranoid symptoms, small doses of anti-psychotic medication might be indicated to dampen down the symptoms of suspiciousness in the early stages of therapy. SSRIs may be indicated for affective dyscontrol and also for lack of impulse control, with the addition of anticonvulsants for the latter.

Producing a Case Conceptualisation or Clinical Formulation

We now turn to the production of a case conceptualisation or case formulation (this will be revisited in the concluding chapter). This seeks to integrate and plan the interventions described above in addition to dealing with the unique narrative that identifies this individual. Case conceptualisation has been usefully defined by Sperry and Sperry [18] as follows: 'Case conceptualisation is a method and clinical strategy for obtaining and organising information about a client, understanding and explaining the client's situation and maladaptive patterns, guiding and focusing treatment, anticipating challenges and roadblocks and preparing for successful termination' (p. 4). It is useful to parse this definition to see how it might apply to someone with ASPD. First, one must *obtain and organise information about the patient*. We have suggested that PD checklists where the criteria are operationally defined are helpful in this respect. This will encompass not only the personality traits of ASPD but also other personality disorders as well. For instance, individuals with ASPD who also have significant paranoid traits will have specific fears (e.g., fears of being taken advantage of) which prevent them from engaging interpersonally. Someone with borderline traits will fear being rejected, excluded or abandoned. Someone with (vulnerable) narcissistic traits will fear social criticism and loss of self-worth. Similarly, it is essential to document any syndromal disorders (especially substance misuse) as any such co-occurrences are likely to hamper progress.

The second task is **to understand and explain the patient's situation and maladaptive patterns**. Here it is important to realise that the assessor needs to take into account the individual's life circumstances as well as any personality difficulties together with what motivates an individual to behave as they do. We believe that those with ASPD believe that only they can achieve their aims by depending on the self by whatever means and that this trumps any capacity to relate to another or achieve any meaningful intimacy. In addition, we have seen in Chapter 5 that those with ASPD are typically living alone, impoverished and likely to be educationally disadvantaged. This increases their sense of having to depend solely on themselves in order to achieve any material gain. In addition, these educational disadvantages need to be considered in the construction of any treatment plan as there is little point in someone producing written homework, if, for instance, they are functionally illiterate.

The third component is **guiding and focusing treatment**. As we have seen, for those with ASPD 'troubles come not as single spies but in battalions' so that multiple rather than single problems are the norm. Hence the challenge for the practitioner is not only to identify the appropriate interventions but to sequence these in a rational manner. While every case is different, the following general observations may be helpful: (1) Co-occurring mental illnesses ought to be targeted at an early stage as these are likely to be barriers to any successful progress. (2) If it is to be used at all, medication ought to be used sparingly but may well have a function in lowering anxiety or paranoia at an early stage and hence may be considered as an intervention at that time. (3) Skills-based training is generally non-confrontational and hence (a) it does not increase anxiety and (b) it can be provided by professionals with appropriate skills but who are less costly to employ than those with more experience. This is an important consideration when budgets are limited.

Anticipating challenges and roadblocks (within the therapeutic process) is the fourth aspect mentioned by Sperry and Sperry [18]. This has especial relevance for those with ASPD. It emphasises that the process of change will not be easy, as those with ASPD have a constellation of maladaptive traits allied to a core belief that one can depend only on oneself; consequently, help from another is viewed not only with suspicion but as a challenge to the individual's core persona. Consequently, managing such conflicts that will inevitably emerge early in the course of treatment is essential if this is to proceed to a satisfactory conclusion. The patient may not initially be aware of the likelihood of such conflicts but it is essential that the therapist is aware of them in advance so that he or she is in a position to deal with them.

In this connection, the work of the late Jeremy Safran with his focus on '*therapeutic ruptures*' is especially pertinent [19]. Briefly, Safran defined such therapeutic or alliance ruptures as 'moments or periods in therapy when there is a strain or breakdown in the therapeutic alliance'. These can range in quality and intensity from a complete breakdown and withdrawal from treatment to a patient sensing that something is wrong in the relationship but choosing to ignore it. They are important in that patients as well as therapists may tend to be unaware of or ignore ruptures. Therapists may also lack the skills to deal with them in a constructive way. Helpfully, Safran provides criteria whereby such alliance ruptures can be identified and suggests a process whereby they can be managed effectively. Rupture markers include, for instance, change in affect, increased irritation with the therapist or decreased involvement (e.g., not doing homework, dropping out of sessions).

When a rupture occurs there is a natural tendency for the therapist to ignore or play down its importance lest they lose contact with the patient. This, in Safran's view, is a mistake since the therapist needs to explore actively the reasons for the rupture occurring by focusing the patient's attention on the event and examining the way in which it is experienced. In an ideal world, the patient explains the experience that is then validated by the therapist. More often than not, however, the patient will deny that the rupture has occurred. Should this be the case, the therapist needs to explore the ways in which the patient avoids recognising and exploring the rupture. Here, it is invaluable for the therapist to have an in-depth knowledge of the maladaptive ways in which the patient has previously handled (or mishandled) similar situations in the past. Clearly, this is a high-wire act and needs to be handled sensitively lest the therapeutic relationship be damaged irrevocably. Nonetheless, the therapist needs to manage such ruptures in a way that will provide essential learning for the patient (i.e., the situation may be fraught but it can be redeemed).

In addition, there are procedures that the therapist can use to reduce the likelihood of such alliance ruptures recurring. These include (1) having a clear therapeutic rationale which is shared with the patient at the outset, (2) agreeing to goals in advance and the tasks necessary to achieve these, (3) respecting the patient's defences and exploring their adaptive function collaboratively, (4) giving and expecting feedback on the therapeutic alliance and allowing the patient to express negative feelings about it and (5) the therapist accepting their responsibility for the alliance rupture (if this seems appropriate). The crucial ingredient is that this is a real relationship that requires give and take on both sides and encourages learning that many conflicts are not black and white but have an element of grey that needs further examination. In this connection, it is important to recognize that either party may fail and come up short. Here, we have found that quoting Samuel Beckett's comment on failure is useful as it contextualizes the experience – 'Ever Tried, Ever Failed, No Matter, Try Again, Fail Again, Fail Better' – and introduces the notion that everyone fails but the essential challenge is to fail better in the future.

The fifth and final component in the case conceptualisation is the **preparation for termination**. It is easy to forget when the initial focus is so much on engaging the patient that disengagement and how this is managed is equally, if not more, important. Holmes succinctly covers the questions surrounding termination (from an analytic perspective) as follows [20]:

> 'The questions surrounding termination are fairly simple, even if the answers less
> so. When should one end – is it up to the analyst, the patient, or when an agreed fixed term is
> 'up'? How should one end – abruptly, or with a gradual winding down of frequency of sessions?
> Are follow-up, and 'top-ups' allowable? Why should one end – what is the theoretical
> justification for an ending, how does one know that the job is done, and how does a decision to
> end emerge?

Holmes points out that while the answers to these various questions are not simple, what is crucial is that the issue is at least thought about. Not thinking about it is perhaps best exemplified by two anecdotes in which termination was not sufficiently thought about and in which one of the authors was actively involved. The first was a practice in which needy prisoners transferred to specialised in-patient services were provided with an intense level of intervention, only for this to end suddenly when they were discharged back to prison with very little if any thought given to their ongoing support. (This has now been sensibly changed with psychologically informed planned environments [PIPES] to support the individual who has returned to prison or to a probation hostel.) Understandably, this abrupt transition from a supportive to a hostile environment was not beneficial.

The second involved a clinical trial and its subsequent replication for personality disordered patients in the community [21, 22]. The design was such that individuals were provided with the intervention for up to for 20 weeks but with nothing offered thereafter. There were two reactions to this abrupt termination. On the first occasion, the patients themselves spontaneously formed their own support group which continued to run for several months without any professional involvement. The second trial – which was a replication of the first – did not have such a benign outcome as the trial had to stop because of the excessive number of adverse events in the active treatment arm [22]. While there was evidence from qualitative interviews with the patients that the active arm of the trial was having a beneficial effect, the planned abrupt termination of the trial caused much distress, resulting in an excessive number of adverse events.

The important message to take from this is that while it is difficult to engage those with ASPD, it is probably more difficult to disengage once a therapeutic alliance has been formed. So how and when the therapy should end needs to be thought about before any intervention takes place. Indeed, the harms caused by a mishandling of the disengagement process could arguably outweigh any benefits that may have accrued from the intervention. Building the 'how' and 'when' of termination into the case conceptualisation directs the therapist's attention to this important component which might otherwise be ignored.

Conclusion

As this chapter has ranged widely over the treatment of those with ASPD, it may be helpful here to summarise some key points. The following are the main take-away messages:

- Good-quality evidence for any specific psychological or pharmacological intervention for those with ASPD is almost non-existent. It is therefore imperative that a sensible and defensible pragmatic guidance to aid the practitioner be produced.
- Non-specific rather than specific factors are important in effecting a favourable outcome in psychotherapy. These include (1) establishing a meaningful and authentic relationship with the patient so that the latter feels that engaging in it will produce positive benefits, (2) creation of expectations that progress can be made and hope is engendered and (3) specific health-promoting actions.
- The role of psychotropic medication is secondary and attention has to be paid to its misuse in this patient group. Nonetheless, we would encourage its use in cases of extreme distress or to facilitate engagement in the early stages of treatment. Concurrently, co-occurring mental illnesses are very common in this disorder and should be actively treated.

- Difficulties in engagement with this patient group because of their personality constellation ought to be seen as the rule rather than the exception. Hence, the therapist ought to anticipate possible ruptures to the therapeutic process and address these proactively.
- Production of a case conceptualisation or clinical formulation at an early stage is essential in knitting together all of these disparate elements. At the same time it must be acknowledged that this will likely require revision in the light of new information becoming available.

References

1. S. Gibbon, N. R. Khalifa, N. H.-Y. Cheung, B. A. Völlm, L. McCarthy. Psychological interventions for antisocial personality disorder. *Cochrane Database of Systematic Reviews* 2020, issue 9, no. CD007668. doi: 10.1002/14651858. CD007668.pub3.

2. N. R. Khalifa, S. Gibbon, B. A. Völlm, N. H.-Y. Cheung, L. McCarthy. Pharmacological interventions for antisocial personality disorder. *Cochrane Database of Systematic Reviews* 2020, issue 9, no. CD007667. doi: 10.1002/14651858.CD007667.pub3.

3. W. J. Livesley. Conceptual issues. In: W. J. Livesley, R. Larstone, eds., *Handbook of Personality Disorders*, 2nd ed. New York: Guilford Press, 2018; 3–24.

4. D. L. Sackett, W. M. C. Rosenberg, A. Muir-Gray, R. B. Haynes, W. Scott-Richardson. Evidence based medicine: What it is and what it isn't. *British Medical Journal* 1966; **312**: 71.

5. D. P. McAdams. Psychopathology and the self: Human actors, agents, and authors. *Journal of Personality* 2020; **88**: 146–155.

6. E. E. Griffith, A. Stankovic, M. Baranoski. Conceptualizing the forensic psychiatry report as performative narrative. *Journal of the American Academy of Psychiatry and the Law Online* 2010; **38**: 32–42.

7. P. R. McHugh, P. R. Slavney. *The Perspectives of Psychiatry*. Baltimore, MD: Johns Hopkins University Press, 1998.

8. National Collaborating Centre for Mental Health (UK). *Antisocial Personality Disorder: Treatment, Management and Prevention*. NICE Clinical Guidelines, No. 77, 2010; www.ncbi.nlm.nih.gov/books/NBK55345/ (accessed 18 December 2020).

9. S. Gibbon, C. Duggan, J. Stoffers, N. Huband, B. Vollm, M. Ferriter. K. Lieb. Psychological interventions for antisocial personality disorder. *Cochrane Database for Systematic Reviews*. Published online 2010. doi:10.1002/14651858.CD007668.

10. N. Khalifa, C. Duggan, J. Stoffers, N. Huband, B. Vollm, M. Ferriter, K. Lieb. Pharmacological interventions for antisocial personality disorder. *Cochrane Database for Systematic Reviews*. Published online 2010. doi: 10.1002/14651858.CD007667.pub2.

11. L. J. Siever, K. L. Davis. A psychobiological perspective on the personality disorders. *American Journal of Psychiatry* 1991; **148**: 1647–1658.

12. M. J. Lambert. The efficacy and effectiveness of psychotherapy. In: M. J. Lambert, ed., *Bergin and Garfield's Handbook of Psychotherapy and Behavioural Change*, 6th ed. Hoboken, NJ: John Wiley & Sons, 2013; 169–218.

13. M. J. Lambert, D. A. Vermeersch. Effectiveness of psychotherapy. In: M. Hersen, W. H Sliedge, eds., *Encyclopedia of Psychotherapy*, vol 1. London: Elsevier, 2002.

14. B. E. Wempold. How important are the common factors in psychotherapy? An update. *World Psychiatry* 2015; **14**: 270–277.

15. H. Glasse. *The Art of Cookery Made Plain and Simple* (1747). Reprint Prospect Books, 1983.

16. M. Zimmerman, W. H. Coryell. Diagnosing personality disorders in the community: A comparison of self-report and interview measures. *Archives of General Psychiatry* 1990; **47**: 527–531.

17. J. Reich, R. G. Vasile. Effect of personality disorders on the treatment outcome of Axis 1 conditions: An update. *Journal of Nervous and Mental Disease* 1993; **181**: 475–484.

18. L. Sperry, J. Sperry. *Case Conceptualisation*. New York: Routledge, 2012.

19. J. D. Safran, J. C. Muran. The resolution of ruptures in the therapeutic alliance. *Journal of Consulting and Clinical Psychology* 1996; **64**: 447–458.

20. J. Holmes. Termination in psychoanalytic psychotherapy: An attachment perspective. In: J. Salberg, ed., *Good Enough Endings: Breaks, Interruptions and Terminations from Contemporary Relational Perspectives*. New York: Routledge, 2010; 63–82.

21. N. Huband, M. McMurran, C. Evans, C. Duggan. Social problem-solving plus psychoeducation for adults with personality disorder: A pragmatic randomised clinical trial. *British Journal of Psychiatry* 2007; **190**: 307–313.

22. M. McMurran, M. Crawford, J. Reilly, J. Delport, P. McCrone, D. Whitham, et al. Psychoeducation with problem solving (PEPS) therapy for adults with personality disorder: A pragmatic randomised controlled trial to determine the clinical effectiveness and cost-effectiveness of a manualised intervention to improve social functioning. *Journal of Personality Disorders* 2017; **31**: 810–826.

Treatment of ASPD, Part 2
Specialist Approaches

Overview

This chapter examines specialist approaches to the treatment of ASPD at a process and at an individual level. At the process level, we consider the phases of personality exploration and integration which can be addressed once emotional stability has been attained by the approaches detailed in the previous chapter. Since these phases make extra demands on the therapist's expertise and competence, the importance of 'fit' between therapist and therapy is examined. It also makes demands on the patient, who needs to have sufficient capacity to engage at this level. The phases of this stage of therapy are described with reference to Livesley's Integrated Modular Treatment.

At the individual level, we focus on the reduction of criminality and violence in those with 'severe ASPD' who may be detained in secure hospitals or incarcerated in prisons. This overlaps with the treatment of psychopathy. The principles of the risk-needs-responsivity (RNR) and Good Lives Model (GLM) are considered and contrasted. Finally, the management of those who are deemed beyond treatment is examined and its implications discussed.

Introduction

We have already pointed out that that the division between generalist and specialist approaches in the treatment of ASPD is somewhat arbitrary. Nonetheless, we believe that this distinction is helpful in structuring our discussion. Furthermore, ASPD is somewhat unique among PDs insofar as its treatment straddles the divide between mental health and criminological interventions. In this chapter we therefore aim to cover treatment from both a specialist mental health perspective and a criminological perspective.

One first needs to consider what resources are available and their likely costs. Hence, while it might be acceptable for a practitioner in a high secure hospital to engage in lengthy and costly therapy with high-risk inmates, this would be an unreasonable expectation to place on a primary care physician. We therefore need to match the severity of the patient's problems with the resources available in such a way that those with the greatest need (which we will define below) are managed by those with the greatest level of expertise. Particularly to be avoided are situations where either (1) those with the highest needs – those who have complex psychopathology or are at high risk of further serious offending – are managed by those with low capabilities, since this is unlikely to end in a good outcome, or (2) those with a low level of need are managed by those with a high level of sophistication, leading to a wasteful use of resources.

Specialist approaches can be considered in one of two ways. First, at a 'task' level, once emotional regulation has been established, intervention extends beyond a 'skills-based' approach to address issues of exploration and change progressing to integration. This corresponds to phases 4 and 5 of Livesley's Integrated Modular Treatment [1], which we shall describe below. Second, the severity of the patient's history and presenting problems can be viewed as markers for the need for more specialist interventions. This especially applies to addressing the criminological needs of the patient. We will first consider more specialist approaches at the 'task' level.

Beyond a Skills-Based Approach: Personality Exploration and Integration

If an individual with ASPD has achieved a degree of emotional stability, one may then consider progressing to interpersonal exploration and integration. This comes with two caveats. First, its suitability needs to be considered carefully since it is likely to increase anxiety in the patient, particularly if the patient lacks the necessary social skills to engage in this process. Second, it is important that the therapist has sufficient skills to manage it. In many ways, whichever form of psychotherapy is chosen – cognitive analytic therapy, mentalising-based therapy, schema-focused therapy, or others – is less important than that the therapist feels comfortable with its principles and processes. This raises the important issue of why so many psychotherapies should exist for the same condition. In the previous chapter we highlighted the importance of the non-specific effects of psychotherapy. Here, we will briefly discuss the importance of the match, not between therapist and patient, but rather between the therapist and the therapy. The importance of this matching has long been recognised in the psychotherapy literature but, to our mind, has been insufficiently emphasised. For instance, Frank & Frank wrote [2]:

> My position is not that technique is irrelevant to outcome. Rather, I maintain that … the success of all techniques depends on the patient's sense of alliance with an actual or symbolic healer. This position implies that ideally therapists should select for each patient the therapy that accords … with the patient's characteristics and view of the problem. Also implied is that therapists should seek to learn as many approaches *as they find congenial and convincing.*
>
> (emphasis added)

This implies that there has to be an adequate match between the therapist and the therapy such that in practising it, the therapist finds the therapy both 'congenial and convincing'. This is hardly surprising since if one is going to spend much of one's life in a particular pursuit, then it surely makes sense that one is comfortable in its principles and practices. This matching is both subtle and rarely discussed, which might explain the tenacious hold that particular modes of therapy have on their adherents. Our observation is that certain therapists are drawn to particular therapies, with some favouring behavioural therapies, some cognitive behavioural therapies, some interpersonal psychotherapies, some psychoanalytic therapies and so on. Whatever the initial attraction – which is probably deep and unarticulated – this allegiance will be challenged (and supported) by a lengthy training, attending seminars with like-minded colleagues and having one's work closely scrutinised by senior trainers. It is therefore not surprising that the end product is someone who is deeply committed to the cause. Inevitably, this process leads to a tribal culture whose members strenuously defend their territory.

We emphasise this as the novice is often faced with choosing among a bewildering array of therapies for the same condition, each with its vociferous adherents, so that the process of choosing between them appears daunting. Here again, it is important to emphasise two crucial points. First, it is the non-specific effects of psychotherapy that account for the greatest variance in the outcome; second, the therapist – of whichever modality – has to be committed to that particular modality in order for it to be successful.

We are therefore agnostic about whichever mode of therapy is chosen, be it psycho-analytic, cognitive or behavioural, in this phase of exploration and integration. This is for three reasons. First, as is evidenced from the systematic reviews cited in the previous chapter, good-quality trials show no compelling evidence in favour of one psychological modality over another in the treatment of those with ASPD. Second, many of the therapies share common elements, as we have previously discussed. Third, we believe that the allegiance of the therapist to the therapy is a significant factor in the success of whichever mode of therapy is chosen. No doubt this position will disappoint those who are devoted to a particular type of intervention, but, in the absence of good data in favour of one intervention over another, we believe that this is a sensible position.

Livesley's Integrated Modular Treatment Model

Having considered these general issues, we will now focus on the task facing the therapist at this stage of the treatment. Livesley covers this aspect of treatment very well in phases 4 ('exploration and change') and 5 ('integration and synthesis') [1]. The former has as its goal 'to explore and change the interpersonal pathology that underlies symptoms and problems, impeding adaptation'. The latter focuses on 'construction of a more integrated self-system' (p. 670). Here we will provide no more than a brief digest of some of the points that Livesley makes.

An over-arching model which Livesley has adapted is Prochaska and DiClemente's Model of Change [3] used with addictive behaviours. This distinguishes the following four treatment phases: problem recognition, exploration, acquisition of alternatives, and generalisation and maintenance. This provides a useful framework in which to develop this discussion.

Stage 1: Problem Recognition and Commitment to Change.

As implied by this heading, once the individual has achieved emotional stability through psychoeducation and skills training, there is now a shift in the therapy to identifying underlying maladaptive patterns of behaviour and inculcating a commitment to changing such patterns. Thus, the therapist's task is to draw the patient's attention to particular problems of which the patient might not be aware and then to encourage the individual to commit to changing these maladaptive patterns.

Stage 2: Exploration

This is an extension of stage 1 in which interpersonal patterns of behaviour are linked together, enabling the patient to see that their 'actions arise from inner beliefs rather than from the actions of others' [1, p. 668]. Further, if these problems can be linked to the developmental processes discussed in Chapter 3, then patients can be helped to construct a historical narrative that makes sense of their lives.

Stage 3: Acquisition of Alternatives

Although it may seem obvious that recognising and exploring problems will lead to change, the process is rarely straightforward. Habitual and maladaptive patterns of behaviour are inevitably difficult to change. Hence, the patient needs considerable encouragement to persist with new patterns of behaviour, even when they do not initially produce the desired result. Here, the therapist uses the therapeutic relationship to maintain and enhance the patient's motivation.

Stage 4: Generalisation and Maintenance

The final stage of this process is that the new behaviours are generalised to everyday living. Here, Livesley makes two important points [1]. First, many of the maladaptive schemas are linked to maladaptive traits that are heritable and stable. He therefore suggests that, rather than attempting to change the individual's maladaptive traits, it may be more productive to modulate their expression by helping them to accept and tolerate their basic personality attributes. He provides a useful practical example in dealing with someone who, as in ASPD, is highly sensation seeking and gratifies their need for stimulation through deviant means such as use of illicit substances, excessive speeding, and so forth, with damaging consequences to the individual and others. Livesley points out that such consequences might be avoided if the individual was able to develop alternative interests such as sporting activities and rock climbing. Second, he points out that the problem lies not so much with the trait as with the rigidity with which it is expressed. Therefore, what is required is a more flexible response. For instance, individuals with paranoid traits who interpret any contradiction of their views with suspicion might be helped if the therapist challenges their interpretation with more benign alternatives.

Integration and Synthesis

The purpose of this final phase of Livesley's system is the synthesis of a new self-structure. Two aspects are especially salient here. First, the individual constructs a new self-narrative. According to Livesley, ' Self-narratives organise experiences into a global account of a person's life that explains who the person is and how she or he came to be this way, by building connections among life experiences, personality features, and behaviour, and how these are related across time' [1, p. 671] Conceptually, Livesley's 'self-narrative' overlaps with McAdams' 'narrative self' which we encountered in Chapters 1 and 2. Second, this needs to be accompanied by a broadening out of the individual's experience such that they take the opportunity of 'getting a life and constructing a personal niche'. This is important as it is accepted that, on account of their condition, those with personality disorder 'live restricted lives with few opportunities for satisfaction and personal growth' [1, p.672]. Hence, the therapist's task is to encourage and enable the individual to gain additional skills, obtain employment, and become involved in a social group. Many of these situations arise opportunistically so that the therapist needs to be alive to their occurrence and to encourage the patient to engage so that their life is enriched thereby. Livesley points out that moving the therapy to this level 'makes the therapy less predictable because the problems and issues raised vary considerably within and between sessions' [1, p. 666]. It therefore makes additional demands on the therapist, who has to be experienced, competent and, if working within a larger framework, affiliated to an organisation that is supportive of the process. In addition, the patient has to have sufficient strength to engage in this process since it will present additional demands and challenges for them.

We illustrate this final phase of treatment in Livesley's model by presenting the following clinical vignette.

Clinical Vignette

Y was a young man in his late teens who was shy and introverted and hence was surprised when a young woman at work took an interest in him. He became infatuated with her and this led him to poison some of his workmates when they made disparaging remarks about her. He was sent to a secure hospital where the same infatuations with some female members of staff recurred. While his initial course was problematic as he was difficult to engage, a careful clinical conceptualisation suggested that the way in which he reacted to others interfering with his infatuations was the result more of emotional turmoil rather than cold-blooded sadistic interest; hence, it was concluded that he might benefit from a suite of psychological interventions. After a long period of various treatments (which included establishing self-control and improving his self-image together with individual psychotherapy with an experienced therapist), Y was deemed to have made sufficient progress to be allowed leave to the community.

Of special relevance here is that Y was a gifted musician and played a number of reed instruments to a high level. He was fortunate in obtaining training in a prestigious course in instrument making and repair which he completed successfully. While on the course, he developed a relationship with another female student, which alarmed his supervising clinical team in the light of his previous history. He reluctantly agreed to disclose his previous history to her (in the presence of a staff member so that details were not minimised). The young woman was unfazed by his disclosure and their relationship continued. A follow-up ten years later revealed that they were still together – each pursuing independent careers – and that he had no further contact with mental health services. In Livesley's terminology he had 'got a life' [1].

The latter part of Y's history, from attending the music course and developing, on this occasion, a satisfactory relationship with a woman, represents a fledgling taking its maiden flight. Inevitably, it raises questions such as: Is this the right time? Am I going to crash on the rocks below or am I going to soar to being independent and free? And the answer, of course, is that you do not know until you – and the system that incarcerates you – has the confidence to allow you to do so. We see that in Y's case, an initial period of chaos and turmoil was followed by a slow maturation (while in secure care), until finally there was a flowering into an autonomous human being. Being able to integrate and establish continuity between these different aspects of the self is important in producing a coherent explanation of 'who the person is and how she or he came to be this way, by building connections among life experiences, personality features, and behaviour, and how these are related across time' [1].

Staff Training and Support

Before considering the interventions for those individuals with ASPD who exhibit violent behaviour and criminality, we will digress briefly here to emphasise some broad principles regarding the provision for those with personality disorder in general and those with ASPD in particular.

Following the publication of the NIMHE document, *Personality Disorder No Longer a Diagnosis of Exclusion* [4], the last two decades have witnessed a more positive approach to the treatment of those with personality disorder in the United Kingdom. This increased interest has not been as productive as it might have been, partly because the document emphasised the need for specialist personality disordered services targeting those with complex needs.

This has led to two unfortunate consequences: (1) a concentration on providing only for those with borderline personality disorder (BPD), as these are the prototypic treatment seekers among those with PD, and a neglect of most of those with other PDs (including ASPD) who do not seek treatment; (2) this limited provision inevitably resulted in long delays in accessing specialist services and several individuals never being deemed suitable for admission. This has left many community mental health teams (CMHTs) with individuals that they do not want and who do not want the services provided for them.

This has led to a reconsideration of the appropriateness of specialist provision for those with PD, with a recommendation that CMHTs ought to be the primary provider with specialist services being involved only in exceptional circumstances [5]. Those with ASPD, particularly if this was associated with violence, would constitute such an exceptional circumstance requiring specialist interventions. This would particularly be the case if there were legal requirements that had to be met. Provisions for such individuals will be considered in the next and subsequent sections. However, it is likely that even these individuals may be in receipt of services from a CMHT at some time in their trajectory, so that these considerations are still relevant. We will now examine some of the organisational and training implications that such a provision would need to establish for it to be successful.

Organisational Structure: It needs to be acknowledged that CMHTs already have a number of advantages in providing for those with PD in general (including those with ASPD). These include the following. (1) They have various skills to deal with a wide range of psychopathology; this is important as many of those with PD will have many comorbid mental illnesses. (2) The stable structure of CMHTs means that the loss of key individuals has less impact on the continuity of an individual's care than if, as in the case of a specialist service, they were dependent on a sole individual. (3) CMHTs' experience of managing those often treatment-resistant individuals with a psychotic illness provides them with a capacity to engage and contain individuals with personality disorder who might also be reluctant to engage. (4) As an intermediary service between specialist services and primary care, CMHTs are in an ideal position to signpost whither and when the individual with PD ought to embark in transitioning between services. (5) Finally, and perhaps most importantly, the condition of some of those with PD may remain chronic. Consequently, a low but lifelong engagement may be necessary, and a CMHT is ideally structured to provide this role.

Training Requirements: While we have made a case for the primacy of CMHTs in the provision of services for PDs in general (including those with ASPD), this process will not succeed without additional resources and training. In the light of the general principles identified in the previous chapter, this will require establishing a therapeutic relationship with the patient by identifying the personality disorder (or disorders) that may be present together with a treatment plan that addresses the individual's difficulties. Simple methods whereby this can be achieved are provided by the simple classification by severity in the new ICD-11 classification. Cognisance needs to be taken of the fact that these are individuals who have multiple problems and contact with multiple agencies, including – in the case of ASPD – with probation, social services, housing and other institutions. Hence the question arises as to how such ancillary agencies ought to be informed by the individual's difficulties. Fortunately, this question has been anticipated by another document of the National Institute of Mental Health England (NIHME) that focused on providing staff with a range of training options to allow them to interact effectively with this group [6]. However, providing interventions in secure settings where those with ASPD may be detained provides particular challenges, which we will now discuss.

The Importance of Treatment Integrity

One of the strengths of the criminogenic approach – the focus of the treatment being the reduction of further criminal behaviour – is that a great emphasis is placed on programme fidelity, the degree to which therapists deliver what they are supposed to deliver. Consequently, close monitoring of the therapist's performance in this regard is built directly into any programme delivery and evaluation. While this approach has undoubted advantages, it has been criticised as being too rigid and formulaic [7]. Notwithstanding this criticism, criminogenic programmes have a great deal to teach those in mental health services about programme integrity.

Coherence and integrity of the approach are critical components when delivering treatment in secure settings. Of necessity, these are complex environments with many factors that may interfere with a coherent delivery of treatment. There may, for instance, be a conflict between security requirements and those of the therapy. If inmates, for instance, are repeatedly searched for security purposes, this does little to engender trust in the inmate. In large institutions, in particular, patients are managed by multidisciplinary teams whose members are likely to spend very different amounts of time with the patient. In psychiatric hospitals, nurses – with varying degrees of training and expertise – are likely to spend a much greater amount of time in direct contact with a patient than a therapist who may visit only once a week. Similarly, in a prison, prison officers will spend more time interacting with an inmate than a visiting therapist.

In order to integrate and resolve differences arising from these differing perspectives (organisational, security, etc.), attention has to be paid to several factors. First, there must be a coherent treatment philosophy that pervades the entire unit; second, staff must be signed up to this and be properly informed; and third, regular multidisciplinary staff meetings must take place wherein differences between staff and between disciplines can be explored and resolved. More often than not, these meetings can become empty rituals where members of the team feel disenfranchised and that they are simply going through a process. Hence, we believe that the organisational heads of the system need to give this due attention. A particularly pernicious issue is that of splitting within the team.

Splitting may arise due to a number of factors. First, a health care professional may have a particularly benign view of a patient as a result of developing a close relationship with them, and this relationship may be challenged by other members of the team. Second, a psychiatrist or psychologist who sees the individual for a single weekly session may similarly have an overly benign view of their patient. This may be challenged by those who have more regular contact and hence a better knowledge of the individual's behaviour across a range of settings

A common problem occurs when the patient discloses something important but prefaces this by saying: 'As I have a good relationship with you and trust you, I am going to tell you this, but it must not be disclosed to others within the team.'

While this should obviously raise alarm bells in the recipient, it is surprising how often these signals are ignored. We emphasise, first, that the philosophy of the unit needs to be embedded in the minds of those who work on it and that it be shared and supported by the wider institution and, second, that it is the duty of senior management to ensure that this is supported through genuine team meetings whose members feel sufficiently confident to speak their mind and believe that they will be listened to. This requires a real effort by the senior members of the team, not only to embed such a culture of inquiry within a clinical team but to maintain it over time. Unfortunately, in our experience what passes for this process is often a tokenistic exercise where there is little or no real engagement among the team members. Engagement of an external facilitator may appear to be an expensive addition, but if they are experienced, sensitive and able to manage the dynamics of the team, they may be an essential item rather than a luxury.

The health of a clinical team may be gauged by its response on occasions when a major breach of security occurs, for example, someone escaping or a staff member having a relationship with an inmate/patient. Inevitably, the clinical team who allowed this transgression to take place, together with the larger employing organisation, has to be called to account. But in our experience the result is an adversarial culture more focused on attributing blame and responsibility than on identifying the causes of the event occurring in the first place. While a healthy team can manage this process and learn from it, it is clearly preferable to avoid this in the first instance.

Dealing with Individuals with Severe Personality Disorder (and Criminality)

We will now consider treatment at the individual rather than at the task level and thereby seek to bring together some disparate areas including the treatment of those at the severe end of the antisociality spectrum and those with psychopathic traits.

A useful starting point is the classic study by Bonta, Law and Hansen, who examined whether the predictors of recidivism were the same among mentally disordered and non-disordered offenders [8]. They found, first, that the major predictors of recidivism were the same in both groups and, second, that while criminal history variables were the best predictors, ASPD was the only clinical variable to have predictive value. It can be concluded that, with the exception of ASPD, the predictors of recidivism in those with mental disorder are related to criminological characteristics rather than to mental disorder.

This study has two implications for practice. First, in order to reduce recidivism, one needs to focus on criminological characteristics. Second, ASPD ought to be considered separately when intervening to reduce further recidivism as its psychological underpinning also needs consideration. Bonta and colleagues' findings are consistent with those reported by Bolaños and colleagues [9]. These authors suggested that, when treating criminal justice–involved persons with mental illness, practitioners should assess and treat not only symptoms associated with their mental illness but their criminal risk as well, in particular, antisocial personality, attitudes toward criminal associates, and job-seeking behaviour.

Those with PD are at increased risk of behaving violently – particularly if the PD is severe and comorbid with other Cluster B PDs [10]. As suggested in this review, the risk of violence appears to be especially high in those with ASPD when paranoid thinking is prominent in the presentation; see Box 7.1.

The association of ASPD with violence was demonstrated in a systematic review and meta-analysis carried out by Yu and colleague [11]. They compared 10,007 individuals with PD with 12 million general population controls. While PD in general was associated with a three-fold increase in risk of violence, the increased risk associated with ASPD was 13-fold. Surprisingly, women with ASPD were more likely to be violent than men with ASPD. In a separate analysis, they found that PD was also associated with repeat offending (OR = 2.4; 95% CI 2.2–2.7).

Available research evidence reviewed by Porter and colleagues indicates a clear relationship between psychopathy and violence, particularly when this is cold-blooded and premeditated [12]. It is clear then that the reduction in violent offending and recidivism needs to be a focus when treating those with ASPD, especially when they show psychopathic and borderline traits. We deal with recent developments in the treatment of psychopathy later in this chapter.

Box 7.1 Clinical Vignette

A defence solicitor requested an assessment of J, a 23-year-old single man who had been charged with the murder of his drug-dealing partner. He had no previous contact with mental health services, although he had served numerous prison sentences for drug possession and violence. He was very guarded at interview, stating that he did not need to be seen by a 'strink' as there was nothing wrong with him; moreover, his partner had got what was coming to him as he was certain that he was skimming on the side. It required a series of interviews to establish any degree of emotional contact and obtain a history. This disclosed that J was the only child of emotionally unfulfilled parents who was constantly denigrated and subjected to physical abuse. He ran away from home at age 11, living rough, engaging in delinquent behaviour, petty thieving, etc. He quickly established himself in the drug trade because of his violence and cunning. While he had numerous one-night stands, he never had any long-term, intimate, sexual relationship as he doubted the fidelity of any sexual partner. In regard to his index offence, he said that, although he had no direct evidence, he had been suspicious that his partner had been siphoning off money from their drug business for some time. When his partner denied this, it only fuelled his belief that he was lying. A fight ensued and he fatally stabbed his partner with a knife. He did not regret his behaviour, saying, 'It's a dog eats dog world out there and if you don't look after number one, who else will?' During the interview, the assessor was conscious that great care was required not to antagonise him as innocuous comments could easily result in being misinterpreted and he would storm out of the room. On specific inquiry, he met criteria for antisocial and paranoid personality disorders. Features of the latter condition included bearing grudges, suspiciousness, reluctance to confide in others, and so on. He refused any offers of help from mental health services as he did not trust professionals and was worried that he might be forced into treatment.

Interventions to Reduce Criminality

Risk-Needs-Responsivity (RNR)

Partly emanating from results of Bonta and colleagues' study cited above, a parallel criminological literature with a focus on reduction of re-offending has developed independently of the literature on mental health. The prevailing view in the 1970s was that 'nothing works' [13]. This pessimism shifted in the 1980s when a view emerged that, in order to reduce recidivism, deterrence via punishment of offenders needed to be supplemented with psychological interventions [14]. The success of the latter was predicated on three principles: first, the risk (R) principle, meaning a focus on high-risk offenders; second, the needs (N) principle, meaning a focus on the assessment and treatment of offenders' criminogenic needs (such as criminal attitudes, substance misuse, impulsivity); and third, the responsivity (R) principle, meaning that the intervention is delivered such that engagement is maximised. The acronym 'RNR' now represents an established process in the rehabilitation of offenders.

The central tenet of this approach is an explicit targeting of whatever criminogenic needs that the individual exhibits with interventions aimed at either reducing or eliminating them. It is important to recognise that features that challenge the therapeutic process (e.g., hostility, poor motivation) are characteristic of high-risk offenders and have to be considered in planning the intervention. The implications of this type of thinking for treatment selection for psychopathy are obvious: 'high-PCL-scoring patients are high risk offenders and should be those most highly prioritized for intensive intervention rather than being considered ineligible for intervention because they are difficult to treat' [15].

Here, it is important to note that mental health abnormalities do not feature prominently in the RNR construct. This is because, as discussed above, mental health abnormalities (with the notable exception of ASPD) contribute little to the prediction of future criminality. Furthermore, RNR is focused on reducing further recidivism of any offender – whether mentally disordered or not – and this has consequences for service delivery.

McGuire provides an apt and positive summary of the impact of the RNR treatment philosophy, saying that 'there is sufficient evidence currently available to substantiate the claim that personal violence can be reduced by psychosocial interventions ... and that emotional self-management, interpersonal skills, social problem solving and allied training approaches show mainly positive effects with a reasonably high degree of reliability' [16]. The alert reader will note that these are the interventions which are much more part of the generalist repertoire discussed in the previous chapter rather than the more advanced psychotherapeutic components of synthesis and integration described by Livesley [1].

The Good Lives Model

The Good Lives Model (GLM) provides a bridge between RNR and the type of process advocated earlier in this chapter. It argues that while RNR is an important approach, it is not sufficiently comprehensive as it focuses too much on the individual's inadequacies. Specifically, with reference to offenders: 'Merely teaching them how to identify their own risk factors and avoid situations where they are likely to engage in harmful behaviours is unlikely to work' [17].

As stated by Ward and Brown:

> The focus (in RNR) is on the reduction of maladaptive behaviours, the elimination of
> distorted beliefs, the removal of problematic desires, and the modification of offence supportive
> emotions and attitudes. In other words, the goals are essentially negative in nature and
> concerned with eradicating factors rather than promoting prosocial and personally more
> satisfying goals. [18, p. 245]

In contrast, GLM rests on the following four principles: (1) it is a strength–based
approach; (2) it views dynamic risk factors as internal and external impediments in the
acquisition of primary human goods (i.e., valued aspects of human living); (3) it focuses
on the necessary skills to engage in treatment (i.e., treatment readiness); and (4) it places
an emphasis on the therapist's attitude toward the offender (and especially on the need to
have a strong therapeutic relationship). Critics of GLM (e.g., [19]) believe that its focus
on non-criminogenic needs might lead to an increase in offending. For instance, Ogloff
and Davis write,

> Until such time that the good lives model can be empirically tested, there is a risk that
> expanding the focus of addressing needs beyond those that are criminogenic may actually
> end up showing no improvement in reducing re-offending. Worse yet, to the extent that
> such rehabilitation efforts may unwittingly lead to the reinforcement of criminality,
> a good lives approach may actually lead, counter-intuitively, to an increase in
> recidivism. [19, p. 237]

Nonetheless, one of the main concerns of RNR critics remains, namely, that by
concentrating on the elimination of various undesirable behaviours rather than promot-
ing positive goals, RNR is insufficiently focused on the issue of the patient's motivation
and engagement. The high rate of treatment non-completion seen among PD patients,
associated with poor treatment outcomes and recidivism [20], is likely attributable in
part to a lack of focus on motivation. This was identified in a recent meta-analysis as
significantly contributing to the high drop-out rates seen in patients with borderline PD
[21]. RNR has been criticised for its emphasis on the primacy of reducing criminogenic
needs, seeing engagement and promotion of health as secondary considerations. For
example, Ziv criticised RNR's advocates for neglecting the role of motivation, stating that
'they ignore the possibility that the internal drive to achieve basic human needs may be
another source of motivation to change criminal behaviour. They are also reluctant to
guide correctional intervention in using motivation for the attainment of offenders'
personal goals, which may enhance their well-being' [22, p. 87].

It appears that advocates and critics of GLM differ in terms of emphasis rather than
real content. Perhaps, more importantly, intervening in those with ASPD (and here we
include psychopathy) acts as a bridge between these two perspectives since, first, it is one
of the few psychological conditions associated with future re-offending [8]; second, as we
saw in Chapter 1, at least 42% of those incarcerated have ASPD and 22% have psychopathy. We turn our attention to the treatment of psychopathy later in this chapter.

Managing Those beyond Treatment and Treatment Failures

It would be remiss in this section not to discuss three thorny issues which most
therapeutic regimes have no need to consider let alone make explicit provision for in
their management. We refer here to clients who are so damaged or have such

characteristics that either they are beyond any intervention or intervention makes the individual worse. Moreover, despite the best endeavours of the treating professionals, the individual either rejects the interventions offered or fails to improve as anticipated. We will now deal with each of these in turn.

Are Some Individuals beyond Treatment?

For anyone who has worked in any branch of therapeutics, the notion that everyone is potentially treatable or that a 'cure' is available for everyone is patently absurd. Nonetheless, we believe that some of those engaged in offering psychological therapies in this arena find it difficult to accept this principle. Clearly, it begs two further questions: First, what are the characteristics of such individuals that can be identified in the first instance? And second, how should they be managed in the long term? We will first address some important questions regarding the treatability of 'psychopaths'.

Are 'Psychopaths' Treatable?

Traditionally, psychopathic individuals were deemed to be untreatable (e.g., [23, 24]. An early study evaluated the impact of a therapeutic community programme on the recidivism rate of 'criminal psychopaths' [25]. This showed that while the programme was effective in reducing violent recidivism among non-psychopaths, it had the reverse effect among psychopaths. The authors of this study later concluded that 'no effective interventions yet exist for psychopaths. Indeed, some treatments that are effective for non-psychopaths actually increase the risk represented by psychopaths' [25, p. 563]. This pessimistic conclusion was challenged in a subsequent systematic review which pointed out the absence of research into the comparison of treated psychopaths with non-treated psychopaths [26]. A more optimistic view has been sustained in recent reviews carried out by Polaschek and Skeem [27] and by Wong [28].

The question of whether 'psychopaths' are treatable can be broken down into five subsidiary questions, as follows:

1. Are psychopathic individuals treatable in principle? (i.e., should a high PCL-R psychopathy score make them ineligible for treatment?)
2. Are psychopaths difficult to treat? (i.e., are there features of psychopathy that make them especially challenging to therapists?)
3. Does a high psychopathy score predict treatment outcome?
4. Can psychopathy itself (as a set of deviant personality traits) be treated? In particular, is there any evidence that traits associated with psychopathy change as a function of treatment?
5. Are psychopathy variants differentially responsive to treatment?

Polaschek and Skeem [27] reviewed the rather meagre evidence pertaining to treatment of adults with psychopathy, which as they point out has relied on the PCL-R to define psychopathy: 'Heavy reliance on these (PCL) scales underrepresents heterogeneity among high-scoring offenders (e.g. differences in anxiety, fearfulness, emotional reactivity) that may have important implications for treatment, and has profoundly confounded the specific personality pathology of psychopathy with general factors related to criminal propensity' (p. 710).

In addressing question 1 above ('Are "psychopaths" treatable in principle?') these authors conclude from a small pool of available studies that a high PCL-R psychopathy score does not present an obstacle to effective treatment to prevent re-offending. Despite not being randomised control studies, in the authors' opinion 'these studies were rigorous enough to challenge lingering beliefs that the risk of commission of new crime by high-psychopathy offenders is impervious to intervention' (p. 713). However, they point out that it is not clear why or how treatment completion leads to reduced reconviction. They state: 'it will be important to show that basic psychopathic tendencies are amenable to change and that these changes relate to improved long-term outcomes' (p. 713).

In addressing the question 'Are "psychopaths" difficult to treat?' the authors answer in the affirmative, pointing out that high PCL scores are associated with a range of negative personality characteristics that are relevant to treatment. For example, they may be angry and irritable, prone to feeling victimised, suspicious of others' motives, antagonistic, aggressive and untrustworthy. Compared with low PCL scorers, high PCL scorers tend to be evasive, verbally combative, hostile, prevaricating, disruptive, less ready to change, less committed to adjunct activities such as work and education, and more likely to leave treatment prematurely. The authors point to the importance of distinguishing between, on the one hand, the therapist's subjective experience of the process of treating psychopathic offenders and, on the other hand, objective measures of the beneficial outcomes of treatment.

The difficulties of treating high-psychopathy individuals is illustrated by two studies. The first examined outcomes in a therapeutic community (TC) treatment program for adult male offenders [23]. Psychopathic offenders, defined by a PCL-R score of 27 or greater, showed less clinical improvement, displayed lower levels of motivation and were discharged from the program earlier than non-psychopaths. The second study [29] focused on inpatient disruptive behaviour in mentally disordered offenders during medium security treatment. It found that interpersonal/affective features of psychopathy (PCL-R Factor 1) predicted a greater likelihood of treatment drop-out. Findings highlighted the importance of a responsive treatment climate in retaining what is a difficult-to-treat group in treatment.

In answering the question, 'Does a high psychopathy score predict treatment outcome?' Polaschek and Skeem conclude from the studies they review that PCL psychopathy scores do not predict treatment outcome.

In addressing the question of whether psychopathy itself (as a set of deviant personality traits) can be treated, Polaschek and Skeem point to a lack of current research that directly addresses this issue. They point out: 'There is certainly value to society in reducing the severity of the underlying personality pathology in psychopathy, if such an aim is achievable' (p. 716). The authors optimistically argue that psychopathic traits may not be intractable.

Perhaps the most important question, so far as treatment is concerned, is the final one: 'Are psychopathy variants differentially responsive to treatment?' Polaschek and Skeem suggest studies should focus on the 'primary' versus 'secondary' variants of psychopathy. We noted in Chapter 4 the important distinction between 'primary' (bold/emotionally stable) and 'secondary' (disinhibited/aggressive) psychopathy variants and the important implications of this distinction for treatment. We noted that whereas primary psychopathy is considered largely ego-syntonic, secondary psychopathy is associated with high levels of dysfunctional negative emotions and comorbid internalizing problems. As such, secondary psychopathic individuals may exhibit greater treatment motivation in order to reduce their own suffering. Primary psychopathic individuals are unlikely to find such treatment targets compelling. Indeed, primary 'psychopaths' are, by virtue of their personality characteristics, more likely to undermine and sabotage any conventional treatment process. Identifying the consequences of their behaviour and the extent to which their choices do or do not support their own self-interests may be more motivationally salient [30].

Polaschek and Skeem suggest that research indicates that psychopathic individuals should be regarded as high-risk offenders – difficult, high-need, complex cases for sure – but not distinctly impervious to treatment. In a similar vein, Wong argues that psychopathy is not untreatable; when focused on PCL-R Factor 2 traits, treatment can be effective in reducing re-offending risks [28]. Complementary to the reduction of future violence arising from PCL-R Factor 2 traits is the need to address behaviours arising from PCL-R Factor 1 traits that may interfere with therapy. In line with the non-specific factors in psychotherapy heavily emphasised in GLM, it is important, Wong suggests, to engage with the offender and to maintain a therapeutic relationship with them. As illustrated by Wong's Violence Reduction Programme, there is therefore a need to incorporate engagement and motivational components that address the Factor 1 (affective and interpersonal) components of PCL-R into any treatment programme for psychopathy. As noted above, in the case of primary psychopaths it will be important to identify factors that are motivationally salient for them, for example, factors that appeal to their self-interest. Conversely, akin to specific factors in our model, criminogenic needs are tackled by specific interventions directed toward reducing the risk of further offending. In practical terms, achieving the goal of reducing recidivism is often deemed a sufficient goal for the forensic therapist.

Polaschek and Skeem [27] point to the need to develop measures of change in core psychopathic traits and to broaden the range of outcomes beyond just recidivism, to address the following questions:

1. Does treatment just reduce criminal behaviour, or does it actually lead to broader reductions in socially and personally harmful behaviour?
2. Does it improve desistance outcomes and increase prosocial behaviour (e.g., participation in employment, decreased alcohol/drug use, more responsible parenting)?
3. Does it set up conditions that may help with community reintegration?

Risk of Recidivism in Sexually Sadistic Offenders

As we saw in Chapter 2, a key characteristic of sadism is that the individual derives pleasure and satisfaction from inflicting harm on others, particularly in the context of sexual coercion (sexual sadism). We also saw that psychopathic features, particularly emotional detachment, meanness and excitement seeking, are characteristic of sexual sadists. As discussed by Longpré and colleagues [31], sexual sadism has traditionally been described as a specific clinical entity, and sadists as individuals who commit serious crimes involving coercion, who suffer from pervasive sexuality disorder and – most important – who present a high risk of recidivism. This has often been invoked to justify harsh punishments such as chemical castration and long prison sentences. Two key questions arise. First, is sexual sadism a feature of psychopathy that adds to the risk of offending over and above other psychopathic features? If the presence of sexual sadism added to the risk, it would clearly be important to identify it, since a failure to do so would put other potential victims at risk. Second, how should such individuals be managed in the long term? This last question applies to psychopaths more generally, and will be considered in a later chapter dealing with legal and ethical issues.

Evidence reviewed by Longpré and colleagues questions the assumption that sexual sadists are at high risk of re-offending [32]. A recent meta-analysis by Eher and colleagues [33] revealed that while sexual sadism may be relevant to an understanding of the severity of sadistic offending, it does not seem to be associated with a higher risk of recidivism. However, Eher and colleagues' meta-analysis showed that the presence of psychopathic traits greatly increases the risk of recidivism among sadistic offenders. Longpré and colleagues conclude from their review of this evidence: 'While a diagnosis of sexual sadism does not automatically mean that the individual has a greater risk of recidivism, its conjunction with the presence of psychopathic traits significantly increases the risk of recidivism' [32, p. 402].

On the basis of the current empirical evidence, Longpré and colleagues argue that the current categorical diagnosis of sexual sadism is problematic and requires re-examination.

Where Offering an Intervention Leads to Harm

This section can be approached by asking two questions: First, what is the evidence that psychological interventions (after all, the staple diet of treatments for those with ASPD) may produce a result opposite to that which is intended? Second, does treating those with severe levels of antisociality, as measured, for example, by a high score on the PCL-R, actually make the offender more likely to re-offend (the reverse effect to that which was intended)? Hence, in this section we will review the evidence that psychological treatments may produce unintended adverse reactions.

Although monitoring an adverse reaction to a drug is commonplace in the prescription of medicines, there is a growing awareness that similar monitoring ought to take place when psychological treatments are administered. After all, any potent treatment may result in an individual getting worse rather than better. Consequently, as psychological treatments become more efficacious, there is a parallel need to consider the 'harm' they may produce [34]. Here, 'harm' is defined as a sustained deterioration caused by the intervention. Such harm may arise from three possible sources: first, from the therapy's adverse effects (e.g., the choice of an inappropriate intervention for the condition or an incorrect application of a correct intervention); second, from features of the patient that make them unsuitable for the intervention; third, from organisational deficits such that provision is suboptimal, for example, large caseloads, inadequate supervision and support of the therapists, and so forth.

Lilienfeld has produced a list of harmful psychological interventions that included Boot Camp Interventions and the Scared Straight Programme for juvenile offenders [35]. The latter involved exposing juvenile offenders to established adult prisoners for a day in a prison with the intention of scaring them sufficiently so that their career trajectories might be changed. As the initial evaluations showed an 80–90% success rate and as this was an inexpensive intervention to administer, it was rolled out through 30 jurisdictions in the United States and further afield. However, a more thorough meta-analysis showed the Scared Straight Programme had the opposite effect to that which was intended; it increased the rate of reoffending by between 1.6% and 1.7% in those exposed to the programme [36].

Another example of a sensible and rational intervention that had unintended consequences is provided by the Cambridge-Somerville Youth Study (1936), again for at-risk juveniles [37]. This intervention sought to remedy the multiple deficiencies faced by disadvantaged youth by providing 'support, friendship and timely guidance' to both the parents and the child by a trained counsellor for five years. In order to apply academic rigour to the experiment, the individuals were first matched and then randomised into the treatment and control conditions. There were a number of follow-ups of this trial at different time periods, and while the individuals and their parents were very satisfied by the intervention, this did not translate into objectively measured improvement in comparisons between the treatment and control conditions. The most enlightening follow-up, however, was that conducted at 30 years by Joan McCord, who achieved an astonishing 98% ascertainment rate [37]. This showed that those in the treatment group fared worse across a range of outcomes. For example, in the 103 pairs where there was a difference, those in the treatment group were more likely, first, to have died prematurely; second, to have suffered from more major mental disorders; third, to have committed two or more crimes; fourth, to have shown signs of alcoholism; and, last, to have lower levels of occupational attainment [38]. One explanation for this unexpected outcome was the influence of deviant peer pressure (the so-called peer contagion effects [39]). The influence of deviant peer pressure assumes greater importance when one considers that many programmes for personality disordered offenders are offered in a group format.

The critical point here is that clinicians need, first, to be mindful of the fact that psychological treatments have the capacity to harm and, second, to be sufficiently alert to detect such harm. The evidence from psychological trials, which is the only place that such evidence is collected systematically, is not encouraging. For instance, the reporting of adverse events in such trials is especially poor in mental health where 'very few drug trials and practically none of the non-drug trials have adequate reporting of clinical adverse events' [40]. Evidence that this applies to ASPD is provided by a review of psychological interventions for personality disorder where adverse events were mentioned in only one of 11 trials [41] and in none of 27 trials for borderline PD [42]. Hence, it is essential that clinicians are aware of the fragility of their patients with ASPD and that they offer interventions only where these are appropriate. As indicated in the previous chapter, termination should be properly thought through in advance.

The Role of Medication

The use of psychotropic medication is not recommended for those with severe personality disorder as, first, there is no good evidence for its efficacy and, second, there is an increased likelihood of abuse. However, its use cannot be totally dismissed. After all, if one is dealing with an extreme end of the spectrum of psychopathology, this may require an extreme solution. Unfortunately, the evidence for such an approach comes only from single reports or small case series and hence carries little weight; nonetheless, this should not be dismissed out of hand. There is evidence, for instance, that in the case of women with borderline personality disorder who engage in extreme self-harming behaviour, clozapine (an antipsychotic medication) has proven to be effective. Evidence in support of the efficacy of clozapine comes from a case series of women in a high secure hospital in the United Kingdom who engaged in extreme self-harming behaviour [43].

We have already referenced the importance of paranoia as a core component of ASPD/psychopathy so it seems logical to consider the use of antipsychotics in those at the extreme end of the ASPD/psychopathy spectrum. A recent report [44] showed beneficial effect of using clozapine in a series of seven men in a UK high secure hospital who were high-scoring psychopaths (i.e., on the PCL-SV, they all scored 19 or above out of 24; mean: 19.6; range: 19–21). These clozapine-treated men showed a major reduction in impulsive, dyscontrolled behaviour and violence. Unfortunately, such a report raises as many questions as it answers. For example, on the basis of such evidence, is it appropriate to administer treatment if the individual does not consent? As ever in this field, high-quality data are lacking so that it leaves the practitioner with a dilemma: Should an intervention be imposed on an individual which might benefit them in the case when they cannot or will not consent, or should treatment be withheld so that they suffer the consequences? This question will be considered further in Chapter 8.

Forensic Case Conceptualisation or Formulation

Although there is considerable similarity between the generic clinical formulation (discussed in Chapter 6) and a forensic case formulation, an important difference must be emphasised. Essentially, a forensic case formulation has as its focus an evaluation of the risk (usually of violence) that an individual exhibits and what might be done to reduce this risk. Hart and colleagues point out the 'process of (such a) formulation is intended to generate an idiographic treatment plan … more than a generic treatment plan such as one based on diagnosis or practice guidelines' [45, p. 118]. Thus, while many of those given a forensic case formulation are likely to meet the criteria for ASPD, the diagnosis is not important. In addition, forensic case formulation recognises the uncertainty attached to many of the predictions given the absence of good data and strong theories. Hart and colleagues state: 'We simply cannot with precision, predict what will happen to patients in the future or, with certainty, calculate what treatments will be most effective for them' [45, p. 119].

This again ought to temper our confidence, not only in the certainty of risk prediction but also in the interventions that might reduce it. A forensic case formulation might be underpinned by a variety of methodologies, but structured professional judgement (SPJ) is currently favoured by most experts [46].

Conclusion

As this and the preceding chapter make clear, intervening in those with ASPD, particularly if psychopathic features are present, is by no means straightforward. Not only does ASPD exhibit a wide range of severity with correspondingly different treatment objectives, but a bemusing variety of interventions is available. These can be used singly or in combination, and in varying degrees of concentration. It is not surprising, therefore, that the therapist may be confused when deciding on a possible treatment plan.

As with other branches of therapeutics, the absence of good-quality evidence from properly conducted randomised trials results in confusion when selecting possible interventions for those with ASPD. Unfortunately, this situation is likely to continue in the short term, and while we would encourage rigorous evaluation of existing and new interventions, this inevitably will take time. Hence, in the absence of any major break-throughs in the near future, what sensible advice can one now offer the practitioner in the management of those with ASPD? Here, we underscore the importance of the following general principles:

- We have already emphasised that it is the general rather than the specific factors that are important in explaining the variance in the outcome of psychological interventions for those with PD in general. There is no reason why this should not apply to those with ASPD. As there appears to be little difference in outcome between the different psychological interventions, an important consideration is that the therapist is comfortable with the therapy.

- The administration of the therapy ought to follow a sequence beginning with engagement, proceeding to establishing emotional control and hence to a revised self-structure. As in the previous chapter, a careful case conceptualisation or formulation is essential so that the purpose of the intervention is shared, not only with other members of the clinical team but with the patient as well.

- Interventions ought to be carefully thought through at an early stage, taking account of the fragility of the individual's psyche together with the organisation's capacity to deliver the intervention. It is imperative that a clear and explicit treatment strategy is adopted and – particularly in forensic psychiatric and correctional settings – the various professionals likely to be involved commit to the strategy.

- Recognising that those with severe personality disorder, particularly where psychopathic features are salient, present a significant therapeutic challenge, the objective of the intervention may need to focus more on risk reduction than on significant personality change.

- Given those with ASPD are likely to misuse psychotropic drugs, pharmacological interventions for those with ASPD should be used sparingly, if at all. Nonetheless, we believe that there is a case to be at least considered when the benefits of intervening are balanced against the rights of the patient to refuse an intervention.

Although those with ASPD are a challenging group to treat, they have considerable treatment needs. Given the damage that they can inflict, not only on themselves but on those close to them and on society generally, the impact of any successful intervention is likely to be considerable. Hence, despite the challenges and failures, it is worth persevering with efforts to improve therapeutic outcomes. We believe that the principles summarised above will provide the practitioner with a rational and defensible mode of practice.

References

1. W. J. Livesley. Integrated Modular Treatment. In: J. Livesley, R. Larstone, eds., *Handbook of Personality Disorders*, 2nd ed. New York: Guilford Press, 2018; 645–675.

2. J. D. Frank, J. B. Frank. *Persuasion and Healing: A Comparative Study of Psychotherapy*, 3rd ed. Baltimore, MD: Johns Hopkins University Press, 1993.

3. J. O. Prochaska, C. C. DiClemente. Stages and processes of self-change of smoking. *Journal of Consulting and Clinical Psychology* 1983; **51**: 390–395.

4. National Institute for Mental Health in England (NIMHE). *Personality Disorder: No Longer a Diagnosis of Exclusion. Policy Implementation Guidance for the Development of Services for People with Personality Disorder.* 2003.

http://personalitydisorder.org.uk/wp-content/uploads/2015/04/PD-No-longer-a-diagnosis-of-exclusion.pdf.

5. C. Duggan, P. Tyrer. Specialist teams as constituted are unsatisfactory for treating people with personality disorder. *BJPsych Bulletin* 2021 (in press).

6. National Institute for Mental Health in England. *Breaking the Cycle of Rejection: The Personality Disorder Capabilities Framework.* Leeds: NIMHE, 2003. http://personalitydisorder.org.uk/wp-content/uploads/2015/06/personalitydisorders-capabilities-framework.pdf.

7. C. Duggan, Why are programmes for offenders with personality disorder not informed by the relevant scientific findings? *Philosophical Transactions of the Royal Society B: Biological Sciences* 2008; 363: 2599–2612.

8. J. Bonta,, M. Law, K. Hansen. The prediction of criminal and violent recidivism among mentally disordered offenders: A meta-analysis. *Psychological Bulletin* 1998; 123: 123–142.

9. A. D. Bolaños, S. M. Mitchell, R. D. Morgan, K. E. Grabowski. A comparison of criminogenic risk factors and psychiatric symptomatology between psychiatric inpatients with and without criminal justice involvement. *Law and Human Behavior* 2020; 44: 336–346.

10. R. Howard. Personality disorders and violence: What is the link? *Borderline Personality Disorder and Emotion Dysregulation* 2015; 2: 12. doi:10.1186/s40479-015-0033-x.

11. R. Yu, J. R. Geddes, S. Fazel. Personality disorders, violence, and antisocial behavior: A systematic review and meta-regression analysis. *Journal of Personality Disorders* 2012; 26: 775–792.

12. S. Porter, M. T. Woodworth, P. A. J. Black. Psychopathy and aggression. In: C. J. Patrick, ed., *Handbook of Psychopathy*, 2nd ed. New York: Guilford Press, 2018; 611–634.

13. R. Martinson. What works? Questions and answers about prison reform. *The Public Interest* 1974; 35: 22–54.

14. D. A. Andrews, J. Bonta. *The Psychology of Criminal Conduct*, 1st to 5th eds. Cincinnati, OH: Anderson, 1994–2010.

15. D. L. Polaschek, J. L. Skeem. Treatment of adults and juveniles with psychopathy. In: C. J. Patrick, ed., *Handbook of Psychopathy*, 2nd ed. New York: Guilford Press, 2019; 710–731.

16. J. Maguire. A review of effective interventions for reducing aggression and violence. *Philosophical Transactions of the Royal Society B: Biological Sciences* 2008; 363: 2577–2597.

17. T. Ward, C. A. Stewart. Criminogenic needs and human needs: A theoretical model. *Psychology, Crime & Law* 2003; 9: 125–143.

18. T. Ward, M. Brown. The good lives model and conceptual issues in offender rehabilitation. *Psychology, Crime & Law* 2004; 10: 243–257.

19. J. R. P. Ogloff, M. R. Davis. Advances in offender assessment and rehabilitation: Contributions of the risk-needs-responsivity approach. *Psychology, Crime & Law* 2004; 10: 229–242.

20. M. McMurran, N. Huband, E. Overton. Non-completion of personality disorder treatments: A systematic review of correlates, consequences, and interventions. *Clinical Psychology Review* 2010; 30: 277–287.

21. E. A. Iliakis, G. S. Ilagan, L. W. Choi-Kain. Dropout rates from psychotherapy trials for borderline personality disorder: A meta-analysis. *Personality Disorders: Theory, Research, and Treatment.* 2021. Advance online publication. https://doi.org/10.1037/per0000453.

22. R. Ziv. The evidence-based approach to offender rehabilitation: Current status of the RNR model of offender rehabilitation. In: P. Ugwudike et al., eds., *The Routledge Companion to Rehabilitative Work in Criminal Justice.* New York: Routledge, 2020.

23. H. Cleckley. *The Mask of Sanity*, 5th ed. St Louis, MO: Mosby, 1976.

24. R. P. Ogloff, S. Wong, A. Greenwood. Treating criminal psychopaths in a

therapeutic community program. *Behavioural Sciences and the Law* 1990; **8**: 181–190.

25. M. E. Rice, G. T. Harris, C. A. Cormier. An evaluation of a maximum security therapeutic community for psychopaths and other mentally disordered offenders. *Law and Human Behavior* 1992; **16**: 399–412.

26. K. D'Silva, C. Duggan, L. McCarthy. Does treatment really make psychopaths worse? A review of the evidence. *Journal of Personality Disorders* 2004; **18**: 163–177.

27. D. L. Polaschek, J. L. Skeem. Treatment of adults and juveniles with psychopathy. In: C. J. Patrick, ed., *Handbook of Psychopathy*, 2nd ed. New York: Guilford Press, 2018; 710–731.

28. S. Wong. A treatment framework for violent offenders with psychopathic traits. In: W. J. Livesley, R. Larstone, eds., *Handbook of Personality Disorders*, 2nd ed. New York: Guilford Press, 2018; 629–644.

29. I. Jeandarme, C. Pouls, T. I. Oei, S. Bogaerts. Forensic psychiatric patients with comorbid psychopathy: Double trouble? *International Journal of Forensic Mental Health* 2017; **16**: 149–160.

30. M. Sellbom, L. E. Drislane. The classification of psychopathy. *Aggression and Violent Behavior* 2021; **59**: 101473.

31. N. Longpré, J. Guay, R. A. Knight, et al. Sadistic offender or sexual sadism? Taxometric evidence for a dimensional structure of sexual sadism. *Archives of Sexual Behavior* 2018; **47**: 403–416.

32. N. Longpré, J.-P. Guay, R. A. Knight. Sadistic sexual aggressors. In: J. Proulx et al., eds., *The Wiley Handbook of What Works with Sexual Offenders: Contemporary Perspectives in Theory, Assessment, Treatment, and Prevention.* Chichester: John Wiley & Sons, 2020; 387–409.

33. R. Eher, F. Schilling, B. Hansmann, T. Pumberger, J. Nitschke, E. Habermeyer, A. Mokros. Sadism and violent reoffending in sexual offenders. *Sexual Abuse: A Journal of Research and Treatment* 2016; **28**: 46–72.

34. G. Parry, M. Crawford, C. Duggan. Iatrogenic harm from psychological therapies: Time to move on. *British Journal of Psychiatry* 2016; **208**: 210–212.

35. S. C. Lilienfeld. Psychological treatments that cause harm. *Perspectives on Psychological Science* 2007; **2**: 53–70. doi: 10.1111/j.1745-6916.2007.00029.

36. A. Petrosino, C. Petrosino, M. Hollis-Peel, J. Lavenberg. Scared straight programs. In: G. Bruinsma, D. Weisburd, eds., *Encyclopedia of Criminology and Criminal Justice.* New York: Springer, 2014. https://doi.org/10.1007/978-1-4614-5690-2_243.

37. J. McCord. Cures that harm: Unanticipated outcomes of crime prevention programs. *Annals of the American Academy of Political and Social Science* 2003; **587**: 16–30. doi: 10.1177/0002716202250781.

38. G. S. McCord. Forward to crime and family: Selected essays of Joan McCord. In: G. S McCord, ed., *Crime and Family: Selected Essays of Joan McCord.* Philadelphia: Temple University Press; 2007.

39. T. J. Dishion, K. A. Dodge. Peer contagion in interventions for children and adolescents: Moving towards an understanding of the ecology and dynamics of change. *Journal of Abnormal Child Psychology* 2005; **33**: 395–400. https://doi.org/10.1007/s10802-005-3579-z.

40. P. N. Papanikolaou, R. Churchill, K. Wahlbeck, J. P. Ioannidis. Safety reporting in randomized trials of mental health interventions. *American Journal of Psychiatry* 2004; **161**: 1692–1697. doi: 10.1176/appi.ajp.161.9.1692.

41. S. Gibbon, C. Duggan, J. Stoffers, N. Huband, B. A. Völlm, M. Ferriter, K. Lieb. Psychological interventions for antisocial personality disorder. *Cochrane Database of Systematic Reviews* 2010; **6**: CD007668.

42. J. M. Stoffers, B. A. Völlm, G. Rücker, A. Timmer, N. Huband, K. Lieb.

Psychological therapies for people with borderline personality disorder. *Cochrane Database Systematic Reviews* 2012; **8**: CD005652.

43. M. Swinton. Clozapine in severe borderline personality disorder. *The Journal of Forensic Psychiatry* 2001; **12**: 580–591.

44. D. Brown, F. Larkin, S. Sengupta, J. L. Romero-Ureclay, C. C. Ross, N. Gupta, M. Vinestock, M. Das. Clozapine: An effective treatment for seriously violent and psychopathic men with antisocial personality disorder in a UK high-security hospital. *CNS Spectrums* 2014; **19**: 391–402.

45. S. Hart, P. Sturmey, C. Logan, M. McMurran. Forensic case formulation. *International Journal of Forensic Mental Health* 2011; **10**: 118–126. doi: 10.1080/14999013.2011.577137.

46. S. D. Hart, C. Logan. Formulation of violence risk using evidence-based assessments: The structured professional judgment approach. In: P. Sturmey, M. McMurran, eds., *Forensic Case Formulation*. Chichester: Wiley-Blackwell, 2011.

Legal and Ethical Issues in ASPD and Psychopathy

Experience should teach us to be most on our guard to protect liberty when the government's purposes are beneficent. Men born to freedom are naturally alert to repel invasions of their liberty by evil-minded rulers. The greatest dangers to liberty lurk in the insidious encroachment by men of zeal, well-meaning but without understanding. [1]

Overview

This chapter explores the legal and ethical issues associated with the involuntary detention of offenders with antisocial personality disorder/psychopathy for treatment in either a secure hospital or prison. It will (1) chart the recent history and changing attitudes toward the compulsory detention of such individuals in the United Kingdom, (2) examine critically the notion of treatability and risk prediction as these are the two main determinants of such a process and (3) conclude with making some recommendations on how such individuals should be managed in the future.

Introduction

In 1996, Dr Lyn Russell, together with her daughters Megan and Josie, were attacked, tied up and savagely beaten with a hammer. Josie was the only survivor, although she suffered brain damage. Naturally, there was considerable pressure on the police to find the perpetrator, and the police did get their man (Michael Stone) a year later from information disclosed by his psychiatrist [2]. Although the only evidence offered by the prosecution was from an informant with questionable credentials, Stone was convicted of a double murder and given two life sentences with a tariff of 28 years.

As Michael Stone had previously been detained in a psychiatric hospital with a personality disorder but discharged as he was thought to be untreatable, this caused considerable angst within the Tony Blair government at the time with its Home Secretary (Jack Straw) declaring, 'It was quite extraordinary that psychiatrists would only take on patients regarded as treatable' (see **Appendix Note 1**).

The conjunction of the horrendous nature of the Russell killings together with officialdom's dissatisfaction with forensic psychiatrists' response to such cases caused the UK government to initiate the Dangerous and Severe Personality Disorder (DSPD) programme.

Despite government support and significant investment, the DSPD programme was subsequently abandoned and replaced with a pathway programme that relied much more on the criminal justice system, with health playing only a minor role. It is also worth noting that Michael Stone, 24 years in to his prison sentence, still proclaims his innocence.

The implementation of the DSPD programme encapsulates several elements that we shall explore in this chapter; to understand this episode properly, it is essential to provide some background so that this policy initiative is properly contextualised.

First, it is important to point out that all patients have a right, with very few exceptions, to refuse medical treatment offered to them and that this applies even when professionals consider that this is not in their best interest. Lord Donaldson expressed this clearly when he affirmed, 'Prima facie every adult has the right and capacity to decide whether or not to accept medical treatment, even if a refusal may risk permanent injury to his health and even lead to premature death' [3].

This autonomy does not extend to those diagnosed with mental abnormality. Two considerations bear on this deprivation: (1) the capacity of the individual may be impaired, and (2) the refusal of treatment may be a risk to either self or others. Clearly, both of these considerations are open to interpretation and we shall see later the different weight placed on each of these by different groups with different agendas. A detailed summary of how this oscillation between autonomy and containment played out in revisions of the 1983 Mental Health Act is provided in an article by Pickersgill [4], to which the interested reader is referred for a more comprehensive account.

Psychopathic Disorder within the 1983 Mental Health Act

When the new Mental Health Act was introduced in 1983, its principles were largely regarded as progressive and humane as compared with its predecessor, but its reception was not without controversy. This especially applies to Part 3 (i.e., the Forensic Sections) of the Act – which deals with patients involved in criminal proceedings. Of the four categories identified in Part 3 – mental illness, severe mental impairment, mental impairment, and psychopathic disorder – it is the last that concerns us here. Psychopathic disorder was defined in the Act as 'a persistent disorder or disability of mind (whether or not including significant impairment of intelligence) which results in abnormally aggressive or seriously irresponsible conduct on the part of the person concerned'. In the case of psychopathic disorder, legislators added a 'treatability test', stipulating 'that such treatment is likely to alleviate or prevent a deterioration of his condition'. This had two purposes: first, in cases where patients would not benefit from treatment, to protect them by preventing their compulsory detention in hospital; second, to protect the hospital so that it was not overwhelmed by unruly and unmanageable patients.

As befits a legal definition, that of psychopathic disorder is understandably vague and empirical studies have identified that a sizable proportion detained under this label also suffer from other mental disorders. For instance, Blackburn and colleagues compared high-security patients detained under the Mental Health Act categories of psychopathic disorder and of mental illness using a number of structured assessments to assess personality disorders, psychopathy and other psychiatric syndromes [5]. They found that, with the exception of more lifetime drug abuse and greater lifetime and current psychosis among those within the mental illness (MI) legal category, the presence of personality disorders, psychopathy or other psychiatric syndromes did not distinguish between the legal categories. A large proportion of patients admitted under the MI category were diagnosable with a personality disorder and vice versa. Despite the qualification of the 'treatability test', forensic psychiatrists in the 1980s were reluctant to admit those with a legal designation of 'psychopathic disorder' as they were sceptical about its validity and treatability. Grounds expressed this scepticism well when he wrote:

> The detention of offenders in the legal category 'psychopathic disorder' in special hospitals for treatment raises a number of critical issues. There are doubts about the nature of the disorder; what constitutes treatment; who is 'treatable'; the effectiveness of treatment; and whether evidence of psychological change implies reduced risk of reoffending. [6, p. 474]

This scepticism was merited as, although the legal category 'psychopathic disorder' clearly contains a heterogeneous group of individuals, the existence of the Special Hospitals Case Register, where long-term clinical and follow-up data were collected, allowed researchers to chart the course of such individuals after their discharge. Such studies produced some influential findings that contributed to professionals' thinking about the treatability and long-term course of this group of individuals. We will describe the findings from three such studies by way of illustration.

In the first study, Reiss et al. [7] applied the PCL-R and DSM-III-R to 89 'young men with a legal categorisation of Psychopathic Disorder' detained at Broadmoor Hospital and examined their institutional behaviour. They found that a PCL-R score of 25 or above was associated with a diagnosis of borderline, antisocial and narcissistic personality disorders, a lack of improvement in social functioning, continued need for seclusion or special care, and discharge to a resource in the community rather than to a hospital. This last finding is somewhat paradoxical in that it suggests that downstream lower secure hospitals were less keen to admit such individuals for admission despite (or perhaps because of) their being deemed to have greater levels of need and risk. The authors' conclusions were prescient in light of the subsequent DSPD initiative. They stated: 'These results should encourage the development of different and specific treatment approaches for these men whilst they remain inside Special Hospital. Their continuing treatment needs and the most appropriate discharge route should be carefully considered' [7, p. 297].

Steels and colleagues [8] compared the long-term outcomes following discharge (mortality and their likelihood of obtaining employment and establishing a relationship) of 75 men and 20 women detained under the psychopathic disorder legal category and 70 men and 19 women legally classified as MI. Both groups showed similar mortality rates, which were twice what might have been anticipated based on a standardised mortality rate of 2.1. However, in other respects their outcomes differed. For example, men with psychopathic disorder were twice as likely to be convicted after discharge and four times more likely to be subsequently imprisoned compared with the MI men, but they were also three times more likely to obtain employment and four times more likely to develop a relationship. In other words, their criminological and psychosocial outcomes were discordant. The women overall had better outcomes compared with the men irrespective of their Mental Health Act classification.

Finally, Jameson and Taylor [9] in a 12-year reconviction study of discharges from high-secure care, confirmed that 'people with personality disorder were seven times more likely than people with mental illness to be convicted of a serious offence'. This illustrates the confusion that can arise from the interchangeable use of the legal psychopathic disorder category and the clinical construct of personality disorder. In the Jameson and Taylor reconviction study, patients followed up were legally defined as having a psychopathic disorder, but their conclusion refers to (unspecified) personality disorder.

In summary, the literature of the 1980s and 1990s led clinicians to have a pessimistic view of the outcome of those with psychopathic disorder. Taylor [10] summarised this well when she wrote that 'follow-up studies consistently show that if the special hospitals confined themselves to the admission and treatment of the mentally ill they could bask in the glow of success, but both the mentally subnormal/impaired and those with psychopathic disorder damage apparent success by the frequency of their re-convictions.'

It was, perhaps, understandable that the 'treatability test' was used by psychiatrists as much to protect the institution and their own reputation as to protect the patient against unlawful detention. One of the concerns therefore was that through its application certain patients were denied the benefits of possible treatment. Hoggett expressed this concern as follows: 'Although the treatability test was introduced to protect the patient against unlawful admission, many believe that it had the paradoxical consequence of excluding patients from care that might otherwise benefit them' [11].

Revision of the 1983 Mental Health Act

In addition to dissatisfaction with certain aspects of the 1983 UK Mental Health Act in the late 1980s and 1990s, there were two additional considerations at play. First, the thinking within government became focused more on the protection of the public and less on the rights of the patient. Second, mental health practice had changed substantially, with a greater emphasis on treating patients in the community and a significant reduction in in-patient beds. Consequently, there was a problem of patients with psychotic illnesses in the community who refused to comply with antipsychotic medication after their discharge from hospital. Legislators therefore sought to plug this gap by introducing compulsory treatment in the community.

In an attempt to resolve these complex and conflicting issues, the government set up an expert advisory committee under the chairmanship of Professor Ginevra Richardson to make recommendations on revision of the 1983 Mental Health Act. One member of the committee later described its remit as follows: 'However, one policy objective was stated with remarkable clarity, and presented as a central tenet critical to the whole programme of reform. That objective was the need for the Committee to address the issue of compulsory treatment in the community' [12, p. 1].

Despite the government's imperative mentioned above, the committee's recommendations, published in 1998, extended further the progressive aspects of the 1983 Act with a greater emphasis on a patient's capacity and autonomy [13]. This was to be followed a couple of months later by the publication of the government's Green Paper on the reform of the 1983 Act, the tone of which directly contradicted the recommendations from its own expert committee [14].

Jill Peay, a member of the Richardson committee, provided a useful commentary on these two documents, laying out their contrasting positions as follows: 'The tone of the two documents is also markedly different, with Richardson's emphasis on non-discrimination, patient autonomy and capacity and the Green Paper focusing on risk as being a, if not the, key factor on which compulsion should turn' [12, p. 8].

Despite the Green Paper's claim that people with mental illnesses 'should be treated in the same way as people with any other illnesses', Peay states that 'it then goes on to advocate criteria for compulsion that are so broadly drawn that it is almost impossible to conceive of an individual who is suffering, or has suffered, from mental disorder who would not fall within the proposed criteria' [12, p. 8]. The Green Paper criticised Richardson's emphasis on capacity as follows:

> The principal concern about this approach is that it introduces a notion of capacity, which, in practice, may not be relevant to the final decision on whether a patient should be made subject to a compulsory order. It is the degree of risk that patients with mental disorder pose, to themselves or others, that is crucial to this decision. [12, p. 35]

It is clear therefore that as far as the government was concerned, risk trumped capacity in the formulation of policy.

In her conclusion, Peay struck an ominous note as regards the DSPD programme when she wrote:

> Finally, it is worth observing that should the Green Paper be adopted in its present form, whatever resolution there is of the current debate over dangerous severe personality disorder (DSPD) will be redundant. For under the Green Paper's proposals, where there is no treatability criterion, there will be no impediment to admitting those with personality disorder and detaining them indefinitely on the grounds of risk. [12, p. 13]

It is this programme's concept and course that we must now examine.

Dangerous and Severe Personality Disorder (DSPD) Programme

The DSPD project (also known as 'the English Experiment') is a useful case study in which various competing issues, discussed below, can be examined. Before considering this, we need to make a brief detour to mention the Dutch TBS system since this in many ways influenced the DSPD proposal. The Terbeschikkingstelling (TBS) literally means 'making a person available for psychiatric treatment'. Within the Dutch criminal code, a TBS order combines a prison sentence with a penal hospital order for treatment in forensic psychiatric (TBS) hospitals. For a judge to impose such an order, the following conditions must be met: (1) The defendant must have a mental disorder (which is ascertained by a psychiatric examination of the suspect), resulting in the responsibility for the crime being (severely) diminished or absent; (2) the crime, typically one that involves violence, carries a prison sentence of at least four years, or the offence belongs to a category of offenses specifically mentioned in the law as carrying a lesser sentence; and (3) there is a risk to the safety of other people or to the general safety of persons or goods [15]. Although the generic term 'mental disorder' is used, studies of the population detained under the TBS order have shown that the vast majority (c. > 80%) meet the criteria for personality disorder [16, 17].

What happens in most instances is that the convicted offender first serves a prison sentence and is then transferred to hospital for treatment. It is important to note that the TBS order is of indefinite duration and involves the involuntary admission to a specialized (high-secure) forensic psychiatric hospital. Consequently, those offenders who are unwilling to engage in treatment, or who do engage but the treatment proves to be ineffective in reducing their risk, potentially face a lifetime of indefinite detention, and this is partly on the basis of their 'mental disorder'. This has subsequently been operationalised within the TBS system so that if an individual has not responded to treatment within six years, then further treatment is abandoned and the individual continues to be detained in a humane way within a psychiatric hospital with no pretence that treatment is being offered. While the imposition of a Dutch TBS order is within the criminal code, such an order can be enacted only when a psychiatrist determines that the individual has a 'mental disorder'. We regard this blurring of the boundaries between criminal justice and health to be problematic for two reasons. First, we regard it as both discriminatory and stigmatising to indefinitely detain someone when this is predicated on the presence of a mental disorder. Second, it rests on questionable risk-driven assumptions.

We return now to the DSPD programme. The impact of singular events (in this case the Russell killings) on public policy should not be underestimated, since politicians need to respond to media and public clamour. We acknowledge, however, that additional factors were at play in instigating the DSPD programme. For instance, recognising that a small number of offenders are responsible for a disproportionate number of offences [18], the identification and targeting of such offenders with effective interventions to reduce subsequent offending could form the basis of a sensible policy. Severe personality disorder (SPD) was one such candidate. For instance, a Home Office policy document identified such a group: 'people with severe personality disorder, who because of their disorder pose a risk of serious offending' [19]. This then became part of a political credo. For example, on page 5 of the UK Labour Party's manifesto in 2001 it was proposed to deal with 'the most dangerous offenders of all, those with a severe personality disorder' [20]. Finally there was, as already mentioned, the government's dissatisfaction with psychiatrists choosing to admit (mostly psychotic) patients for treatment while excluding those with personality disorder.

DSPD allowed for the preventative detention of those who fulfilled the following three criteria: (1) being dangerous, defined as posing a 'significant risk' (>50%) on two risk assessment tools (the duration of this risk being unspecified); (2) having a severe personality disorder (which was defined in various ways); and (3) a link being established between (1) and (2) [21]. Among the consequences of this initiative was the indeterminate detention in hospital of prisoners who met these criteria after they had completed their prison sentence. They were incarcerated not because of what they had done, but what they might do in the future. Not surprisingly, this initiative provoked considerable concern, not only among mental health professionals who were now charged with carrying out the programme, but also from individuals who were so detained.

The government in turn fought back, arguing not only that the initiative was necessary to protect the public but that it provided interventions for those who hitherto had been denied any treatment. This could hardly be contested as very few secure hospitals admitted patients with the legal designation of 'psychopathic disorder'. High-secure hospitals were the exception, although here fewer than a quarter of those detained had a legal designation of 'psychopathic disorder' [9] and moreover this proportion had declined significantly by the 1990s. The contrast with other psychiatric services was stark, with the figure dropping to 'a mere 0.24% among patients compulsorily admitted ... to ordinary NHS facilities in England and Wales' [22, p. 1581]. The hazards of detaining such individuals for 'treatment' were well recognised and included uncertainty regarding the diagnosis, the efficacy of any interventions, and the substantially increased likelihood of further reoffending after discharge. Hence there were understandable reasons why mental health professionals might wish to exclude patients with personality disorder from treatment. On the other hand, there was a groundswell of opinion among mental health activists that this was an opportunity to address the prior neglect of mental health services in the community for those who suffered from personality disorder. This neglect was addressed by the publication of a policy document entitled 'Personality Disorder, No Longer a Diagnosis of Exclusion' [23] together with a training programme to increase workforce capacity in the management of personality disorder [24]

Resolving these various conflicting policy objectives was never going to be easy, but in the teeth of professional and patient misgivings, the DSPD programme was put in place with significant resources devoted to both secure hospital and prison settings. This established that provided an individual met the DSPD criteria, he (initially it was limited to only male offenders but later broadened to include females as well) could be compulsorily detained for 'treatment' in a prison or hospital whether he agreed to have this treatment or not.

Before dismissing this as a gross infringement of an individual's rights (which we believe the initiative was), it is only fair to state some positive features of this initiative. Among the advantages was an explicit underpinning using accepted risk assessments and diagnostic criteria. Unlike their vague legal predecessors, the use of accepted risk assessments and diagnostic criteria at least allowed for proper scrutiny and scientific follow-up to determine the efficacy of intervention(s). There was also generous provision in specialised settings together with funding for much needed research in this area [21]. This included an examination of the effectiveness and cost effectiveness of this new policy [25]. Conversely, there were some major downsides to the DSPD programme. Perhaps most egregiously, in dismissing the individual's capacity to act as an autonomous agent, it also placed mental health professionals more in the role of gaoler than of helper. While the entry criteria were an improvement on the previous Mental Health Act category of psychopathic disorder, all were open to criticism. First, the diagnostic entry criteria appeared to be arbitrarily chosen. Second, the risk assessment tools employed were of doubtful accuracy, particularly in regard to the risk that an individual might pose. Added to this was the fact that it was the criminological characteristics, rather than the personality traits, that accounted for the future risk of criminal behaviour. Finally, the most contentious issue of all was the need to establish a 'functional link' between the presence of the disorder and the risk of violent behaviour. This is discussed further below. Finally, there were questions regarding the efficacy of the treatment programmes employed with little systematic effort made to compare them.

These concerns, together with the government's own funded evaluations that showed the initiative to be a failure (and a costly failure at that) led to a change in strategy such that resources were now directed toward establishing a pathway for offenders with personality disorder within the prison/probation system with health playing only a very minor role [26]. We might also remind the reader of the case of Michael Stone, who continues to proclaim his innocence, having already spent 23 years in prison. The Criminal Cases Review Commission has refused to refer his case back to the Court of Appeal.

Despite its failure, the DSPD programme encapsulated two general issues which we now consider in greater detail: (1) entry criteria and (2) treatability. In this discussion, we restrict ourselves to examining the ethics and legality of compulsorily detaining offenders with personality disorder for treatment in mental health settings. We will not consider other aspects such as offering psychiatric testimony in capital murder charges with the possibility of the death penalty or the indefinite detention of sexually violent predators (SVP in the United States). Concerns regarding use of the PCL-R in such settings are discussed by Edens and colleagues [27, 28].

Entry Criteria

To be compulsorily detained within a mental health facility, the individual (1) needs to suffer from the disorder in question, (2) must exhibit serious risk of harm to self or others, and (3) there must be a demonstrable 'functional link' (i.e., a causal relationship) between the disorder and the risk. We have already mentioned problems associated with the legal designation 'psychopathic disorder' as it was defined in the 1983 Mental Health Act. A step change occurred in the 1980s with the introduction of DSM-III ASPD and Hare's PCL-R measure of psychopathy, which appeared to place the diagnosis of offenders with personality disorder on a firmer footing [4]. Reflecting this thinking, various combinations of these criteria were used as criteria for entry into the DSPD programme. As we have outlined in various places in this book, substantial problems attach to these PD constructs, not least of which is that both conflate personality deviation with criminality. Hence, one cannot have confidence that these criteria are sufficient to meet the test of accuracy that might be expected when individuals are to be detained against their will.

The second consideration involves the risk posed to self and others. While the risk to self in this population is not to be dismissed (see Chapter 5), it is the risk to others that was foremost in assessors' minds when evaluating individuals for compulsory detention. The field of risk assessment has undergone major developments over the past two decades. There is a consensus that clinical judgement – the central tenet of such assessments up to the 1980s, shown to be no better than chance [29] – should be replaced by a more structured approach. While there are a number of risk assessment instruments available, research has shown that there is little to choose between them in the prediction of future dangerousness [30]. While structured risk assessments increase the accuracy of risk prediction over clinical judgement, there remain concerns about the applicability of group data to an individual case (discussed further below). Furthermore, it must surely be a concern that it is the criminological rather than the personality features that are predictive of future violence, although personality features are employed as criteria to justify compulsory detention [30].

A final consideration concerns the third criterion for entry to the DSPD programme: the 'functional link' between (severe) PD and high risk of violence. The current authors have discussed at length the challenge of establishing a 'functional link' between personality disorder and the risk of further violence [31]. To briefly summarise our critique, we argued that establishing a causal connection in the behavioural sciences (e.g., does severe personality disorder cause violence?) requires that the following criteria be fulfilled: (1) covariation must be demonstrated between the variables; (2) the causal variable (PD) must be shown to temporally precede the onset of violent behaviour; (3) in particular, the possibility that the observed covariance is due to causal operation of a third variable must be excluded; and (4) it must be possible to establish a logical connection between PD and violence, including a specification of possible causal mechanisms to address the question 'How does PD cause violence?' Examination of the evidence suggested to us that the criteria for establishing a causal link between PD and violence had not been met. We argued that the concepts of ASPD and psychopathy were too broad-based and that it was necessary to drill down to more elemental aspects of these broad constructs in order to understand the link between PD and violence risk. A review of the evidence suggested *emotional impulsiveness* and *paranoid thinking* as likely candidates in this regard [32].

Although it is considered to be more rigorous and to have greater predictive accuracy than DSM ASPD, use of the PCL-R as a risk instrument presents particular problems. First, we should note that the PCL-R was never intended as an instrument to assess risk. Second, while a high PCL-R score of between 25 and 30 is perhaps the most acceptable marker of severity in this group, its reliability is limited by not being normally distributed [33]. Third, it is a dubious practice to use total PCL-R scores to make predictions of violence risk, since the PCL-R total conflates criminological variables (mostly in Factor 2, unstable and antisocial lifestyle) with personality deviation (mostly in Factor 1, interpersonal and affective features). A detailed analysis of the ability of individual PCL items to predict violent reconvictions in men following their release from prison showed that only three items (i.e., criminal versatility, poor behavioural controls, lack of stimulation/boredom), all from Factor 2, were significant predictors [34]. None of the Factor 1 items predicted risk of violent reconviction. Another troubling issue is that PCL scores have demonstrated an effect of courtroom adversarial allegiance, with scores being inflated by assessors who were acting for the prosecution [27]. Further, certain Factor I items such as grandiosity, callousness and remorselessness were especially susceptible to inter-rater disagreement [27]. In a thoughtful review of the use of psychopathy assessments in applied forensic settings, Edens and Truong recently concluded [28, p. 23]:

> Courts should examine questions of admissibility more critically than they have in the past, particularly given extant findings that (a) cast doubt on the reliability of PCL-R ratings and ASPD diagnoses in applied (and particularly adversarial) settings and (b) raise significant concerns about the potentially unduly prejudicial effects of introducing such evidence in criminal and civil commitment cases.

Despite the evidence that psychopathic individuals are more likely to engage in antisocial behaviours, these authors caution against the assumption that a particular examiner's evaluation of any given defendant, respondent or prisoner is by definition 'reliable and valid'.

In addition to these considerations, there is a more fundamental objection to the use of risk instruments. The data used to justify a decision to detain an individual on the basis of their risk necessarily come from group data from representative samples, while the task for the risk assessor is to apply such data to an individual case. Attempting to use actuarial risk measures to predict any individual's likelihood of being violent in the future is fatally flawed by the high margins of error observed at the individual level [35]. Faigman and colleagues described this dilemma succinctly when scientists offer opinions in a legal arena, but the same applies in a clinical setting: 'Whereas scientists almost invariably inquire into phenomena at the group level, trial judges typically need to resolve cases at an individual level' [36, p. 417].

Translating from group to individual data is what clinicians do every day in their clinical practice. The challenges in doing so are significant but they do indicate that caution is needed in the interpretation of such a prediction (e.g., some have argued that confidence intervals surrounding reported scores were a more defensible method of reporting results than discrete scores in the PCL-R [27]). A proper development of this area would require a chapter in itself. Let us conclude that a probabilistic rather than a binary answer to a question such as 'Does this person meet the criteria for psychopathy?' is a more sensible way forward.

In summary, there are major concerns in regard to the entry criteria in compulsorily detaining offenders for treatment. While it has been improved, the assessment diagnosis remains problematic, with major questions remaining about the diagnostic status of both ASPD and psychopathy. Similarly, the second component of the entry criteria (i.e., risk) appears to be equally problematic given concerns in regard to its reliability, its accuracy in eliciting core psychological features (as compared with criminological characteristics), together with the difficulty of applying group data to an individual case. Perhaps the most problematic element of the entry criteria is the third criterion: the necessity to show a functional link between severe PD and high risk – in other words, a causal link must be demonstrated.

Treatability

We turn now to the second component required for entry to the system, 'treatability'. A useful frame for discussing this is provided by a seminal paper by Paul Applebaum on 'Psychiatry's Problematic Responsibility for the Control of Violence' [37]. Here, he advanced the notion of reciprocity as the essential element distinguishing 'patients' from prisoners in preventative detention as follows: 'Unlike prisoners in a pure preventative detention system, patients committed to mental health facilities receive direct benefits from their detention beyond those in society at large might derive.' This implies that the patient gives up their freedom, albeit involuntarily, in the expectation that some form of effective treatment will be offered in return. Interestingly, this same principle appears to underpin the Richardson Expert Committee's proposals (see [12, p. 10]). This principle helps to distinguish such incarceration from punishment within the criminal justice system. Applebaum developed this further by specifying three criteria that would need to be met in justifying psychiatric preventative detention: (1) the detention ought to be limited to those patients who are treatable in the setting in which they are detained, (2) the treatment must be provided and (3) patients ought to be detained only as long as the treatment is provided [37] (see Appendix **Note 2**). It follows from (1) and (2) that when clinicians detain a patient for 'treatment', they must be satisfied not only that patient is 'treatable' but that the necessary treatment is both available and effective. Further, (3) above implies that the patient may be detained only for as long as is necessary to deliver the treatment. Once this has been completed, the patient should be released, and this is irrespective of the risk that they might pose.

The first two of these issues was played out in the case of *R* v. *Canons Park Mental Health Review Tribunal, ex parte A*. The following is a brief précis (it is more fully discussed in Baker and Crichton [39]). This involved patient A, who had a history of depression, deliberate self-harm and alcohol misuse, being initially detained under the legal category of mental illness, which was subsequently changed by her Responsible Medical Officer (RMO) to 'psychopathic disorder'. In doing so, he indicated that the 'treatability test' was satisfied since he believed that she would benefit from psychotherapy offered in a group setting. A stated that since she refused to attend group therapy, it followed that she was 'untreatable' and should be discharged. While a Mental Health

Review panel refused to grant her release, a subsequent judicial review found in her favour with Justice Sedley stating that 'it was never appropriate under the provisions of the 1983 Act ... for a patient to be detained in hospital for treatment for psychopathic disorder if he or she is not at that point treatable'. His judgment was subsequently overturned by the Court of Appeal where Lord Justice Kennedy, one of the three judges, argued that 'there was evidence before the tribunal ... that ... a prolonged period of treatment, consisting at first of no more than nursing care and persuasion to accept group therapy, followed by group therapy itself was likely to prevent a deterioration in the patient's condition even if at first some deterioration could not be avoided' [40].

It is interesting to note that that in the 2007 Mental Health Act legislation [41], the 'treatability test' was broadened in scope to include an 'appropriate treatment test' where (in Section 145(1)) treatment is defined as including 'nursing, psychological intervention and specialist mental health habitation, rehabilitation and care'. To us, this gives professionals an extraordinary degree of latitude in determining what constitutes 'treatment'. This inevitably raises concerns that individuals might be coerced into treatment. The fear is that such patients detained in hospital for 'treatment' could easily find themselves in a Catch-22 situation where their detention will obviously continue if they admit the need for further treatment. However, a refusal to take part in treatment may be interpreted as indicating a lack of insight that might require a further period in hospital. It is clear from the foregoing that there are major concerns as to how the 'treatability test' is interpreted. While we have made the case in Chapters 6 and 7 that there is some therapeutic optimism for those with ASPD/psychopathy, this is contingent on there being effective engagement between the patient and both the therapist and the broader organisation. Hence, compelling an individual to accept treatment, or at least to remain in a secure therapeutic facility until such time as 'insight' is gained and acceptance is finally achieved, is not the way forward.

Aside from the detrimental effect on the individual so detained, there is another consideration that is often overlooked, namely, the toxic effect that a treatment-rejecting individual might have on a ward milieu such as in a secure hospital or prison. Group therapists speak of a delicate balance to be struck between the health of the group – which, though not exclusively, is provided by the staff and some of the more mature patients – and the malign and disruptive influence of more severely affected patients (and perhaps some staff members as well). It is considered essential that in order to maintain the health of the group, the balance has to be tilted so that the health component outweighs its malign opponent. The presence of patients who refuse to engage in any activities and are overtly disruptive or dismissive of the therapeutic activities that are on offer are likely to have a very corrosive effect on the culture of a ward.

In summary, the use of personality disorder as a rationale for maintaining public order is unlikely to succeed, not only on account of the objections cited above but also because of the inability of authorities to provide services for those so detained. That said, this debate of balancing public safety against individual liberty is not going to go away and we have to recognise that there are a number of different actors – each with competing agendas. As these are rarely congruent, some disagreement is inevitable. While not wishing to minimise this, we believe that articulating each of these perspectives is more likely to lead to a successful resolution. We will therefore describe these different players and their respective constituencies as a first step to seeking a resolution.

First, there are the **therapists** who would like to effect positive change in a difficult population. Here, there is a natural temptation to admit patients who are compliant and easy to treat, as this will produce better outcomes and provide a more manageable population. As we saw in Chapter 7, well-resourced therapeutic efforts ought to be directed toward those at highest risk, so that admitting compliant and easy-to-treat patients is hardly the best use of resources. Moreover, within multidisciplinary teams there is unlikely to be a consensus, as each member is operating from a different professional standpoint arising from their training and experience. For instance, psychologists are likely to view the 'treatability' of an individual more favourably, and social workers are less keen on the compulsory detention of individuals. Conversely, psychiatric nurses who have to interact with and manage such individuals on a daily basis are less likely to be favourably inclined. The psychiatrist is somewhere in the middle, having to wrestle with these competing opinions as well as being ultimately responsible if anything untoward occurs in regard to the eventual outcome. Hence, managing the dynamics in a multidisciplinary team with these competing interests is challenging.

Second, there are the **government policymakers** who have to wrestle with the competing demands of health (e.g., 'why are we not providing interventions for those in the community with PD who are being denied services?') and justice (e.g., 'why are we not able to protect the public from "dangerous psychopaths"?'). History shows us that justice usually trumps health in such a debate, especially when something horrendous occurs. When there is public and media pressure for 'something to be done', it is understandable that this may result in a hasty decision that may have long-term, damaging consequences. The introduction of the DSPD initiative is one such example. Despite aspiring to base the proposal on evidence, the 1999 Home Office report acknowledged that the process of incarceration could not 'be delayed until the outcomes of research are known' [21]. Here, one has some sympathy with policymakers as research inevitably takes time, while civil servants and their political masters are often forced into a position where an immediate decision must be taken.

Third (and most important) are the **patients** who receive treatment at the expense of losing their liberty. It is clear that views here are mixed, so that, as a consequence of their detention, some are provided with interventions which they might not otherwise have been able to access, while others are caught in a system with no possibility of release.

Conclusions and a Way Forward

We conclude that mental health professionals do have some extra competence (compared with the lay person) in determining the individual's capacity both to engage in further violence and to benefit from treatment. However, such competence is marginal, and, with the evidence currently available, its limitations need to be explicitly acknowledged. Given the high uncertainty in regard to both treatment efficacy and risk prediction, we do not believe that the case for the compulsory admission of offenders with personality disorder has been made.

We will make some recommendations to 'square the circle' between the competing demands of public protection and patient autonomy for offenders with personality disorder. But first some general observations are in order. First, we need to recognise the woefully inadequate mental health provision offered to those with personality disorder in general. While the reasons for this are complex, one is that some would question whether it really is the proper business of mental health services to handle PD on account of uncertainty regarding its classification and treatment efficacy. Second, those with personality disorder are a challenging and not particularly rewarding group to manage. In 1988 Lewis and Appleby described the view among psychiatrists that patients with personality disorder were 'manipulative, attention-seeking, annoying' [42, p. 45]. Third, there is the perception, especially among forensic psychiatrists, that in their decision to admit or not admit risky psychopaths, they are 'damned if they do and damned if they don't' [21]. In other words, they will be blamed if they fail to admit someone for treatment and something untoward happens (as was the case with Michael Stone); alternatively, they will likewise be blamed if they admit and subsequently discharge a psychopathic offender and something untoward happens. As we have seen, the likelihood of something untoward happening is substantially increased for this group.

One of the current authors has argued that mental health professionals need some reasonable protection in the light of the uncertainty (and in some cases the likelihood) of something untoward happening [43]. In that work, it was argued that professionals need to be held to account for any professional failings in the delivery of their service (as would be the case with any other service delivery). But this does not give a level of carte-blanche criticism when something untoward occurs that in retrospect appears obvious to the investigator. In other words, professionals ought to be held to account for any failings in delivery and judgement in regard to acceptable standards of service delivery, but they should not be accountable for something untoward happening if this was outside their control. Risk prediction in this area is enormously challenging. As the academic lawyer Alan Dershowitz writes, 'Predictions of human conduct are difficult to make, for man is a complex entity and the world he inhabits is full of unexpected occurrences. Predictions of rare human events are even more difficult' [44, p. 6].

The second deficit that needs to be addressed is the inadequate provision of services, and this applies to the provision of services to those with personality disorder in the community as much as to those who are incarcerated in special hospital or prison. Fortunately, some progress has already been made. For instance, the 2003 policy document of the National Institute of Mental Health England (NIMHE) 'Personality Disorder, No Longer a Diagnosis of Exclusion' [23] challenged the belief that people thought to have personality disorder were not the business of mental health services. While the implementation of this policy has been patchy, it is nonetheless a welcome step forward.

A Pragmatic Proposal for the Management of Offenders with PD

Turning now to the provision of services to mentally disordered offenders, we propose that the provision of treatment should be completely uncoupled from the serving of a prison sentence. Treatment and incarceration should each stand alone and come together only if and when the convicted offender with a personality disorder voluntarily opts for an intervention. We propose that individuals with a personality disorder who are charged with an offence should, provided that they are fit to plead, stand trial as would any other offender. If convicted and given a custodial sentence, this should be served as it would by any other convicted individual. Hence, offenders with personality disorder would be treated as any other offender without the disorder. This would mean that the individual on remand would not be offered a mental health evaluation prior to the trial (unlike the TBS system). Hence, any conviction and sentence would not be influenced by such mental health considerations.

This separation of health and criminal justice provisions has the following advantages. First, it avoids the danger that many prisoners will exaggerate their symptoms in order to get a hospital rather than a prison disposal. We have already described a case in Chapter 6 where an individual fabricated a psychotic illness in order to avoid a prison sentence. While an extreme case, it is not unique. It is all too easy for someone to endorse symptoms of PD in order to gain a hospital disposal. Second, many psychiatrists have had the experience of a patient's enthusiasm for treatment dissipating shortly after their transfer to hospital. This leads to uncertainty as to what the next step should be. Finally, and most crucially in the present context, the separation of health and criminal justice provisions avoids indefinitely detaining individuals who remain at high risk and who either refuse or are not responsive to treatment (a hazard which both the TBS and DSPD systems inevitably entail). In contrast, we propose that if convicted and sent to prison, offenders with a PD should be either offered suitable interventions within the prison system or transferred to hospital for treatment in special cases. The choice of opting into such treatment needs to be voluntary so that the patient can make an informed choice once the risks and benefits have been explained – as would be the case with any other medical intervention. We believe that since individuals with ASPD or psychopathy are likely to reject rather than seek treatment, their voluntary rather than coercive entry to treatment is essential to a successful outcome and will, in addition, reduces discrimination and stigma.

Unlike the TBS system where the prison sentence is usually served first and treatment introduced at the end, this system is flexible with treatment being offered whenever it is deemed to be appropriate. We accept that some degree of implicit coercion occurs in such a situation insofar as an early release may be contingent on participation. Unfortunately, this is inevitable.

For such a proposal to work, two conditions are critical. First, there needs to be a significant increase in resources for the prison system. While this may seem like stating the obvious, we believe that the rate of recidivism would be reduced in those discharged to the community if they had undergone a period of treatment to which they had voluntarily agreed. It may therefore prove to be cost effective, despite the increased prison costs [45] (see Appendix **Note 3**). Of equal if not greater significance is that support and treatment in the community should be available for those who are released from custody. All too often we have seen that if the offender is not offered the required level of support on discharge, the significant gains achieved in a custodial institution quickly dissipate once the individual is released. Continuing input from services is crucial given that released offenders face significant challenges as regards accommodation, social support, desistence from substance misuse and so forth. Establishing a care pathway that spans several different levels of security and agencies is essential in our view, and it is important that this has been incorporated into the Offender Personality Disorder Pathway [26].

These principles would apply both to the prison and to secure health services. In the former, while risk reduction would be the primary objective, this would be informed by a greater psychological understanding of the personality of the individual (and this would especially apply to the responsivity component). The secure health service might be reserved for more complex cases, particularly those suffering from several comorbidities.

Summary

- In this chapter, we have examined the complex relationship and competing priorities between the health and justice systems through the lens of compulsorily detaining individuals with personality disorder. We have framed this through investigating changes in mental health legislation over the past 40 years in the United Kingdom. We have paid particular attention to the introduction and fate of the DSPD programme in the UK.
- Three principles underpin the compulsory detention of personality disordered individuals: (1) their diagnosis and treatability, (2) their risk to self or others and (3) establishing a causal link between (1) and (2). We argue that the level of uncertainty surrounding all three principles is such that it would be unethical to compulsorily detain such individuals for treatment. Furthermore, to do so would further perpetuate the stigma and discrimination against an already disadvantaged group.
- We therefore propose an alternative approach whereby the health and justice systems are uncoupled such that prisoners on remand are processed by the latter without any involvement of the health system either pre-trial or subsequent to a conviction. Individuals with mental health vulnerabilities who have been convicted and sentenced to prison would then be assessed at that stage (i.e., post-sentence) and could then volunteer for treatment either in prison or, in special cases, in a mental health facility.
- The success of this approach will require significant further investment both in the provision of therapeutic services in prisons and in the provision of appropriate aftercare in the community.

Appendix

Note 1. On the Michael Stone Case

It is only fair to point out that the inquiry into Michael Stone's case disagreed with this conclusion. Robert Francis QC, who chaired the inquiry, wrote subsequently, 'Mr Stone was not someone who was ignored by statutory services and left to his own devices, Indeed the range of services he received and the intensity with which they were provided was remarkable, particularly given the lack of any real progress with him.' And again, in respect of the response from Forensic Services, he commented that 'the forensic psychiatric service was judged to have provided conscientious and accurate assessments of Mr Stone and offered continuous contact with a skilled community psychiatric nurse. Contrary to some media reports at the time, there was no question of the forensic service refusing to admit Mr Stone to hospital. Indeed they went beyond their remit on one occasion by offering in–patient detoxification when other units were unwilling or unavailable to do so' [2, p. 43].

Note 2. The Fate of Those Detained within the DSPD Programme

Tribilcock and Weaver studied the legal status of 172 DSPD patients and prisoners. The following is a summary of their findings taken from their abstract.

Dangerous and severe personality disorder prisoners were more likely to have been serving indeterminate sentences, while patients admitted to hospital units were more likely to have been given determinate sentences. At admission, the majority of prisoners were in advance of their tariff expiry or parole eligibility dates, while the majority of patients had passed them. Patients previously serving a determinate prison sentence were close to their non parole date (NPD), the date they expected to be released from prison, with 40% of pre-NPD patients found to have less than two weeks to serve. At follow-up 85% of patients originally serving a determinate sentence had passed their NPD. While only three prisoners passed their NPD during the study, all were still detained. These findings suggest that a proportion of patients were 'preventatively detained' within the DSPD hospital units. [38]

Note 3. The Consequences When Policy Is Not Followed by Practice

Here, it is useful to quote the consequences of not providing interventions for those who had been mandated to receive them by the court. This is from a report of HM Inspector of Prisons and HM Chief Probation Officer on the demise of Indeterminate Public Protection (IPP) orders I in 2008. 'This was a perfect storm. It led to IPP prisoners languishing in local prisons for months and years, unable to access the interventions they would need before the expiry of their often short tariffs. A belated decision to move them to training prisons, without any additional resources and sometimes to one which did not offer relevant programmes, merely transferred the problem. By December 2007, when there were 3,700 IPP prisoners, it was estimated that 13% were over tariff. As a consequence, the Court of Appeal found that the Secretary of State had acted unlawfully, and that there had been 'a systemic failure to put in place the resources necessary to implement the scheme of rehabilitation necessary to enable the relevant provisions of the 2003 Act to function as intended'. Rather more pithily, a prison lifer governor told us: "It is as though the government went out and did its shopping without first buying a fridge"' [45, p. 2].

A later Prison Inspector's Report in (2016) showed that 'Some had spent more than ten years above their tariff, many for the Kafkaesque reason that courses that the parole board insisted they had to take before being released were not available to them.'

References

1. R. D. Brandais. *Olmstead* v. *U.S.*, 277 U.S. 438 (1928) (dissenting), 1928.

2. R. Francis. The Michael Stone Inquiry – A Reflection. *Journal of Mental Health Law* 2007; 41–49.

3. Lord Donaldson, M.R in Re Adult: Refusal of medical treatment (1992) 4 All E.R. 649.

4. M. Pickersgill. How personality became treatable: The mutual constitution of clinical knowledge and mental health law. *Social Studies of Science* 2012; **43**: 30–53.

5. R. Blackburn, C. Logan, J. Donnelly, S. Renwick. Personality disorders, psychopathy and other mental disorders: Co-morbidity among patients at English and Scottish high-security hospitals. *The Journal of Forensic Psychiatry & Psychology* 2003; **14**: 111–137.

6. A. Grounds. Detention of 'psychopathic disorder' patients in special hospitals: Critical issues. *British Journal of Psychiatry* 1987; **151**: 474–478.

7. D. Reiss, D. Grubin, C. Meux. Institutional performance of male 'psychopaths' in a high-security hospital. *The Journal of Forensic Psychiatry* 1999; **10**: 290–299.

8. M. Steels, G. Roney, E. Larkin, T. Croudace, P. Jones, C. Duggan.

Discharged from special hospitals with restrictions: Psychopathic disorder and mental disorder compared. *Criminal Behaviour and Mental Health* 1998; **8**: 39–55.

9. L. Jamieson, P. J. Taylor. A reconviction study of special (high security) hospital patients. *The British Journal of Criminology* 2004; **44**: 783–802.

10. P. J. Taylor. Special supplement. *Criminal Behaviour and Mental Health* 1992; **2**: iii–v.

11. B. Hoggett. *Mental Health Law*, 3rd ed. London: Sweet & Maxwell, 1990.

12. J. Peay. Reform of the Mental Health Act 1983: Squandering an opportunity? *Journal of Mental Health Law* 2000; 5–15.

13. Department of Health. *Report of the Expert Committee: Review of the Mental Health Act 1983*. London: Department of Health, 1999.

14. *Reform of the Mental Health Act 1983 Proposals for Consultation.* Presented to Parliament by the Secretary of State for Health by Command of Her Majesty, November 1999.

15. C. de Ruiter, R. L. Trestman. Prevalence and treatment of personality disorders in Dutch forensic mental health services. *Journal of the American Academy of Psychiatry and the Law* 2007; **35**: 92–97.

16. C. de Ruiter, M. Hildebrand. The dual nature of forensic psychiatric practice: Risk assessment and management under the Dutch TBS-order. In: P. J. van Koppen, S. D. Penrod, eds., *Adversarial vs. Inquisitorial Justice: Psychological Perspectives on Criminal Justice Systems.* New York: Plenum Press, 2003; 91–106.

17. I. G. H. Timmerman, P. M. G. Emmelkamp. The prevalence and comorbidity of Axis I and Axis II disorders in a group of forensic patients. *International Journal of Offender Therapy and Comparative Criminology* 2001; **45**: 36–149.

18. T. E. Moffitt. Adolescent-limited and life-course persistent antisocial behaviour: A developmental taxonomy. *Psychological Review* 1993; **100**: 674–701.

19. Department of Health; Home Office. *Managing Dangerous People with Severe Personality Disorder.* London: Home Office, 1999.

20. 2001 Labour Party General Election Manifesto 2001. Ambitions for Britain. 2001. http://labourmanifesto.com/2001/2001-labour-manifesto.shtml (accessed 17 December 2020).

21. C. Duggan. Dangerous and severe personality disorder. *British Journal of Psychiatry* 2011; **198**: 431–433.

22. J. Coid, C. Cordess. Compulsory admission of dangerous psychopaths. *British Medical Journal* 1992; **304**: 1582.

23. National Institute for Mental Health in England (NIMHE). *Personality Disorder: No Longer a Diagnosis of Exclusion. Policy Implementation Guidance for the Development of Services for People with Personality Disorder.* 2003. http://personalitydisorder.org.uk/wp-content/uploads/2015/04/PD-No-longer-a-diagnosis-of-exclusion.pdf (accessed 17 December 2020).

24. National Institute for Mental Health in England. *Breaking the Cycle of Rejection: The Personality Disorder Capabilities Framework.* Leeds: NIMHE, 2003. http://personalitydisorder.org.uk/wp-content/uploads/2015/06/personalitydisorders-capabilities-framework.pdf (accessed 17 December 2020).

25. P. Tyrer, B. Barrett, S. Byford, et al. *Evaluation of the Assessment Procedure at Two Pilot Sites in the DSPD Programme (IMPALOX Study).* London: Home Office, 2007.

26. N. Joseph, N. Benefield. A joint offender personality disorder pathway strategy: An outline summary. *Criminal Behaviour and Mental Health* 2012; **22**: 210–217.

27. J. F. Edens, J. Petrila, S. E. Kelley. Legal and ethical issues in the assessment and treatment of psychopathy. In: C. J. Patrick, ed., *Handbook of Psychopathy*, 2nd ed. New York: Guilford Press, 2018; 732–751.

28. J. F. Edens, T. N. Truong. Psychopathy evidence in legal proceedings. In: P.

Marques, M. Paulino, L. Alho, eds., *Psychopathy and Criminal Behavior: Current Trends and Challenges.* Amsterdam: Elsevier Academic Press, 2022, 241–272.

29. J. Monahan. *Violent Behavior: An Assessment of Clinical Techniques.* Beverly Hills, CA: Sage, 1981.

30. M. Yang, S. Wong, J. W. Coid. The efficacy of violence prediction: A meta-analytic comparison of nine risk prediction tools. *Psychological Bulletin* 2010; **136**: 740–767.

31. C. Duggan, R. C. Howard. The 'functional link' between personality disorder and violence. In: M. McMurran, R. C. Howard, eds., *Personality, Personality Disorder and Violence.* Chichester: John Wiley & Sons, 2009; 19–37.

32. R. C. Howard, C. Duggan. Personality disorder and offending. In: G. J. Towl, D. A. Crighton, eds., *Forensic Psychology*, 3rd ed. Chichester: John Wiley & Sons, 2021.

33. D. J. Cooke, C. Michie. Limitations of diagnostic precision and predictive utility in the individual case: A challenge for forensic practice. *Law and Human Behavior* 2009; **32**: 28–45.

34. J. W. Coid, M. Yang, S. Ullrich, T. Zhang, S. Sizmur, D. Farrington, R. Rogers. Most items in structured risk assessment instruments do not predict violence. *Journal of Forensic Psychiatry and Psychology* 2011; **22**: 3–21.

35. P. E. Mullen. Dangerous and severe personality disorder and in need of treatment. *British Journal of Psychiatry* 2007; **190**, S49: S3–S7. doi:10.1192/bjp.190.5.s3.

36. D. L. Faigman, J. Monahan, C. Slobogin. Group to individual (G2i) inference in scientific expert testimony. *University of Chicago Law Review* 2014; **81**: 417–480.

37. P. S. Applebaum. The new preventive detention: Psychiatry's problematic responsibility for the control of violence. *American Journal of Psychiatry* 1988; **145**: 779–785.

38. J. Trebilcock, T. Weaver. Study of the Legal Status of Dangerous and Severe Personality Disorder (DSPD) Patients and Prisoners, and the Impact of DSPD Status on Parole Board and Mental Health Review Tribunal Decision-Making. 2011. Project Report, Ministry of Justice, London.

39. E. Baker, J. Crichton. Ex parte A: Psychopathy, treatability and the law. *Journal of Forensic Psychiatry* 1995; **6**: 101–109.

40. *R v. Canons Park Mental Health Review Tribunal ex parte A* [1994] 2 All ER 659 CA (Law Report).

41. Revision of the Mental Health Act 2007. www.legislation.gov.uk/ukpga/2007/12/contents (accessed 17 December 2020).

42. G. Lewis, L. Appleby. Personality disorder: The patients psychiatrists dislike. *British Journal of Psychiatry* 1988; **153**: 44–49.

43. C. Duggan. Managing personality disorder in the community. In: P. Basant, I. Treasaden, eds., *Forensic Psychiatry.* London: Taylor & Francis, 2014.

44. A. M. Dershowitz. On 'preventive detention'. *New York Review of Books* 1969; 12, 5.

45. HM Chief Inspector of Prisons, HM Chief Inspector of Probation. The indeterminate sentence for public protection: A thematic review. HM Inspectorate of Prisons, September 2008. www.bl.uk/collection-items/indeterminate-sentence-for-public-protection-a-thematic-review# (accessed 17 December 2020).

Conclusions and Future Directions

ASPD as a Diagnostic Construct

In the opening chapter of this book we saw that debate continues about how best to assess and conceptualise PDs. A central, and as yet unresolved, question concerns whether PD categories, and ASPD in particular, should be allowed to survive, or should be jettisoned as has been done in ICD-11. A case can be made for retention of a category-based system of PD assessment on the following grounds. First, clinicians are generally more comfortable dealing with discrete categories or prototypes, which are deeply embedded within the human psyche and are a way of making sense of the world. Westen and colleagues put this well in relation to PD when they wrote that 'recognising a personality syndrome is fundamentally a process of pattern recognition, much as face recognition depends on pattern recognition, not a tabulation of individual features' [1, p. 274]. Second, despite problems concerning their scientific validity, PD categories have been refined over many years and so have what Smith-Benjamin calls 'folk wisdom' [2]. Third, as we argued in Chapter 6, a typology (with its explicit enumeration of relevant traits) can be a useful shorthand for the therapist when engaging the client, particularly when the former is inexperienced and may need a foothold in difficult terrain.

The outstanding question that remains to be addressed over coming years is whether an assessment system that is devoid of PD categories can successfully capture the richness and diverse nature of personality pathology. In the final analysis the dichotomy of PD traits versus PD categories is likely to prove a vacuous one, since both trait (DSM-5 Section 3) and symptom (DSM-5 Section 2) indicators of ASPD (and other PDs) have been found to converge on a relatively coherent construct [3]. The real question is: Does this construct adequately capture antisocial personality? In this book we argue that antisocial personality is much broader than the constructs – psychopathy and ASPD – with which it has traditionally been associated and that new methods are required to assess it. If the clinician finds PD categories useful, they should continue to use them, in the same way that navigators might continue to use the constellations in the night sky without being under any illusion that they represent real objects.

Most work on PD starts from questionable categories of PD (ASPD, psychopathy) and works outward to describe what is often referred to as their 'nomological network' (the network of relations with other measured variables [4]). Contrary to this, our starting point should arguably be *antisocial outcomes*, ranging from petty crime and substance abuse to interpersonal violence and sexual sadism. Starting from these antisocial outcomes one should work backward, first to examine how an outcome such as violence can be parsed motivationally and emotionally (e.g., What emotion goals are being promoted? What value goals are aspired to?) and then to examine how particular motives and emotions are related to personality variables.

If the diagnostic construct of ASPD is to be retained, it will need to be refined since, as currently operationalised in DSM-IV/5, it conflates personality variables with criminality. The result is that, as we saw in Chapter 1, contact with the criminal justice system exerts a disproportionate influence on an ASPD diagnosis. The same criticism can be levelled at the way psychopathy is operationalised in the PCL-R. While the PCL-R has been extremely useful in stimulating research, it has probably outlived its usefulness by perpetuating the misconception that psychopathy is a global entity. As Lilienfeld and colleagues cogently argued, 'psychopathy is not monolithic, therefore etiological efforts would be better invested in understanding the sources of the specific subcomponents of this condition and the mechanisms underpinning their interactions rather than to psychopathy as a global entity' [5]. Consistent with this argument, findings suggest that specific PCL-R items, but not the total score, are predictive of important outcomes. For example, only three PCL-R items, among them need for stimulation/proneness to boredom, were found to predict violent reconvictions in 1,353 men following their release from prison [6]. None of the 'interpersonal/affective' features of psychopathy (PCL-R Factor 1 items, asterisked in Box 1.1 in Chapter 1) was able to predict violent reconvictions.

Models of mental disorders should arguably focus on *symptoms* (and individual traits) rather than on flawed diagnostic *syndromes*: compared with these syndromes, symptoms have more defined boundaries, less heterogeneity, and greater stability [7]. Consistent with this, evidence suggests that particular outcomes – a diagnosis of alcohol use disorder (AUD), number of AUD symptoms, and alcohol consumption – are linked to specific symptoms of PD (impulsivity and affective instability) *independently of their link to PD categories* [8]. In another study, just two diagnostic criteria – impulsivity from borderline PD and childhood conduct disorder (CD) from ASPD – outperformed the full ASPD and BPD diagnoses in predicting AUD [9]. Research suggests that it is specifically *antagonistic traits* within the broad constructs of psychopathy and narcissism that explain their positive relations with aggression and antisocial behaviour outcomes [10].

Taken together, results of these studies imply that to get a clear view of how ASPD and psychopathy are related to negative outcomes, it is necessary to drill down to more elemental aspects of these categories. An example of how this might be achieved was demonstrated in a recent study that analysed self-report personality data obtained using the Dimensional Assessment of Personality Pathology – Basic Questionnaire (DAPP-BQ) from a large sample comprising community subjects and outpatients [11]. Their analysis enabled the authors to decompose a broad 'dissocial behaviour' domain into four facets (callousness, rejection, conduct problems and stimulus seeking), with each facet comprising between four and five sub-facets. Callousness comprised sub-facets of *cruelty, egoism, mercilessness, lack of empathy/guilt* and *utilization/exploitation*. Rejection comprised sub-facets of *dogmatism/intolerance, judgemental attitude, pugnacity* and *bossiness/dominance*. Conduct problems comprised sub-facets of *interpersonal violence, alcohol abuse, theft/illegal behaviour, juvenile violence* and *contempt for norms*. Stimulus seeking comprised sub-facets of *recklessness, impulsivity, sensation seeking,* and *unplanned behaviour*. The dissocial domain was additionally correlated with suspiciousness (comprising sub-facets of persecutory ideas, hypervigilance and distrust) and narcissism (comprising sub-facets of need for approval, fantasies of success and attention seeking). The authors expressed the hope that by describing traits at this (sub-facet) level of detail, it might be possible to achieve more exhaustive and fine-grained assessments and more precise treatment plans. Such a fine-grained assessment would help in providing a more nuanced case formulation, described further below.

We should note that since symptoms represent the actual concerns of clients, it is more appropriate to focus on them from an ethical point of view: each symptom is a valid and important aspect of the client's difficulties that we should aim to understand [7]. A personalised (idiographic) approach to assessment (outlined below), where the patient's individual symptoms are explored and understood, is ethically preferable to a traditional (categorical) assessment. This is because, due to its intensity and depth, a personalised assessment uniquely allows the patient to feel deeply understood [12].

We now briefly consider three aspects of antisocial personality – boredom proneness, paranoia, and revenge – that we consider among its key elements.

Boredom Proneness

Boredom proneness refers to individual differences in the extent to which boredom is experienced more or less intensely, more or less frequently, and – perhaps most importantly – *the extent to which individuals experience their life in general as boring* (see [13] for a useful review). Being boredom-prone will have motivational consequences, since adaptive goal-directed activity depends on an ability to bring our thoughts, feelings and actions in line with our goals, an ability that is compromised in those who are boredom-prone [14].

In two culturally disparate samples, one from the United States and the other from Hong Kong, boredom proneness was reported to be significantly associated with self-reports of anxiety, depression, stress and low life satisfaction [15]. These authors suggested that a global perception of one's life as boring might be related to a lack of meaning, purpose and direction in life (LMPD), discussed further below. We suggest an important distinction might be drawn between two motivationally distinct types of boredom. One, associated with psychopathy (see Box 1.1), reflects a *need for stimulation* and a desire to engage in high-arousal activities in the pursuit of excitement. The other boredom type, most clearly associated with borderline PD and (as we saw in Chapter 4) with vulnerable narcissism, reflects the experience of *emptiness*, an omnipresent and profound feeling of detachment at the intrapersonal, interpersonal and existential levels of experience [16]. Recent findings highlight not just the importance of emptiness as a diagnostic marker for personality pathology but also its usefulness for classifying mental disorders more generally, in particular, internalizing disorders involving self-dysfunction and detachment [16].

How these two sub-types of boredom may be related to ASPD is unknown since there is little evidence about boredom's role in ASPD per se. Insofar as it overlaps with psychopathy, ASPD is likely to be associated most clearly with the boredom type that reflects a need for stimulation. However, emptiness is also likely to be a feature of those with ASPD who present with comorbid internalizing disorders. Boredom is likely to be a particular problem for those individuals in whom ASPD is combined with borderline symptoms, since they would likely suffer from both types of boredom. Motivationally, such individuals would be doubly compromised. On the one hand, driven by a quest for excitement, they will seek out opportunities in their environment that offer the prospect of satisfying their desire for high arousal. On the other hand, having an aversion to social engagement they will avoid opportunities for social interaction. It is perhaps not too difficult to imagine that, caught on the horns of this dilemma, such an individual might opportunistically and impulsively seek self-gratification by engaging with a socially inappropriate but available target, for example, a child.

A contemporary view [17] posits that boredom is associated both with poor self-knowledge and a high degree of self-directed attention. The latter is said to exist in either of two modes: a *ruminative* (anxious/neurotic/inhibited) motivational style or a *reflective* style in which there is a reflective relationship with self. It is proposed that the ruminative mode is associated with a protracted state of boredom from which it is difficult to exit. If this view is correct, it suggests that the boredom experienced as emptiness/lack of meaning in those with internalizing disorders may reflect an excessively ruminative self-focus, and that these individuals may have great difficulty escaping from a protracted state of chronic, unrelieved boredom.

Paranoia

Broadly conceived, paranoia encompasses perceptions of social reference and hostility, suspicious thoughts and mistrust of others, and fears of persecution. In the general community, paranoia is reported to be associated with the risk of having any PD but most robustly with borderline PD [17]. Paranoid beliefs, for example, expectations that others are untrustworthy, duplicitous, and intend to exploit and harm, were found to distinguish UK prisoners diagnosed with ASPD from those not so diagnosed [18]. We should note here that the high rates of paranoia found in incarcerated individuals may, in part, be attributable to the aversive nature of the environment in which they find themselves. Recent findings suggest that paranoia, like psychopathy (as discussed in Chapter 2), is associated with altered patterns of social reward [19]. Specifically, individuals showing greater paranoia reported that they enjoyed positive, prosocial interactions *less* and negative social interactions (engaging in harmful or callous behaviour) *more*. In other words, paranoia was associated with a preference for being cruel over being kind. Evidence reviewed by these authors suggests that paranoia shares similar developmental antecedents and psychosocial correlates (childhood maltreatment, poverty and low socioeconomic status) to those we have described, in Chapters 3 and 5, as being associated with antisocial personality. In Chapter 2 we saw that paranoia can be considered part of an expanded 'dark traits' construct. In short, therefore, paranoid thinking should be considered an important aspect of antisocial personality, broadly conceived, that, in combination with emotional impulsiveness, may account for it being associated with violence.

A systematic review and meta-analysis [20] demonstrated that, in both clinical and non-clinical samples, paranoia is associated with an interpretation bias characterized by *a consistent tendency to interpret emotionally ambiguous stimuli, situations, or events in a negative manner.* Thus a paranoid individual might interpret the stare of a stranger as malicious and threatening. This implicates involvement of paranoia in the impulsive, aversively motivated type of violence shown in Figure 2.4, where the emotion goal is self-protection/safety. Anxiety was found to mediate the association between interpretation bias and paranoid beliefs in patients with distressing paranoia [21]. This suggests paranoia may be a salient feature of the thought disorder attributed, in Figure 2.1, to the personality pathology subsumed under the 'anxious-inhibited' umbrella.

Revenge

The desire to avenge a perceived injustice should not, in itself, be considered pathological. When it maintains self-esteem and restores a psychological balance, an act of revenge can arguably be regarded as a healthy way of coping with insult or injury [22]. However, when the desire for vengeance is long-lasting and becomes dysfunctional in the context of a mental disorder, it can be considered a maladaptive way of dealing with the distress occasioned by a perceived wrong. In this context it may eventuate in a violent act of revenge.

Pathological revenge linked to violent offending was exemplified in a review of 62 cases of revenge filicide [23]. In over half of the cases reviewed, there was an active mental disorder of any type, most often a personality disorder, and most commonly ASPD. The authors of this study pointed out that the acts of revenge filicide reviewed by them often involved significant premeditation and planning; that is, they were often not carried out impulsively. These premeditated acts of revenge are examples of what, in Chapter 2 (see Figure 2.4), were referred to as retributive acts of violence motivated by the emotion goal of vengeance. One subtype ('rejection') among the 62 cases, where the offender was abandoned or spurned by their partner, comprised a substantial minority (39%) of all cases [23]. Figure 9.1 illustrates a plausible mechanism through which rejection may trigger hostile rumination in individuals with personality disorder. Once triggered, a self-perpetuating cycle or 'emotional cascade' [24] of increasing rumination, paranoia and negative affect is set in motion, leading ultimately to commission of a retributive act of violence. Figure 9.1 illustrates that paranoia interacts reciprocally with hostile rumination – the tendency to harbour ill feelings of resentment and a desire for retaliation and vengeance in response to self-threatening provocations [25]. Experimental evidence supports a role for rumination in maintaining paranoid thinking [26].

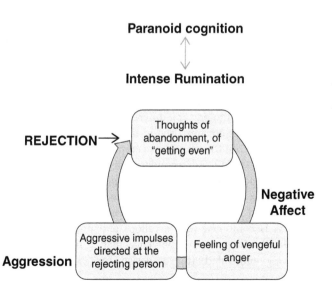

Figure 9.1 An emotional cascade, triggered by rejection, leads to intense rumination which, through a positive feedback loop, serves to increase the intensity of the negative emotion (feelings of vengeance) and aggressive impulses.

The Importance of Motivation

Throughout the various chapters of this book, we have emphasised the importance of considering the motivational and emotional determinants of antisocial personality, in regard to both its assessment and its treatment. Indeed, it is the construct of motivation that links together the treatment-oriented chapters of this book and the more theory-based and research-oriented chapters. At the end of Chapter 1 we outlined a social/motivational model of PD which, consistent with PD essentially reflecting interpersonal dysfunction, emphasises particular motivations for maladaptive interpersonal engagement and disengagement. We reviewed evidence in Chapter 2 suggesting that antisocial individuals, particularly those with high levels of psychopathic traits, lack the motivation to engage in an empathic way with others. We argued that antisocial individuals differ from others with regard both to their *emotion goals* (the emotions that they desire) and their *value goals* (the values that they find desirable). Evidence reviewed there also suggests that, viewed through the lens of a hierarchical model, antisocial personality transcends particular diagnostic categories, reflecting an antagonistic and hostile interpersonal style. Importantly, *antisocial personality is much broader than the constructs – psychopathy and ASPD – with which it has traditionally been associated, with interpersonal antagonism, callousness and hostility lying at its core.*

Developmental Origins

Personality disorders have their origins in childhood and adolescence. In Chapter 3 we saw that a cascade of developmental derailments and insults, from early psychosocial adversity and traumatic brain injury, through academic failure and exposure to deviant peers, to early drug and alcohol abuse, leads to a trajectory of life-course-persistent antisociality. Adolescence was emphasised as a critical period when personality development can be diverted from a prosocial to an antisocial track. We emphasised in particular the importance of excessive substance use in adolescence as a critical factor in derailing normal development and impairing brain function. We outlined two possible gender-linked developmental pathways leading from childhood and adolescence to adult antisociality, one predominantly male, the other predominantly female.

Neurobiology

In Chapter 4 we reviewed the role of neurobiological factors in antisocial personality. We emphasised that a brain and behaviour approach can provide useful clues regarding causation of antisociality. However, describing the latter in terms of abnormal brain structure or function simply re-describes pathology at a different (brain) level. It should not be so surprising if deviant personalities are mirrored in deviant brain structure or function: funny people have funny brains! In this chapter we emphasised the distinction between 'primary' (emotionally stable or 'bold') and 'secondary' (disinhibited/aggressive) variants of psychopathy, which has important implications for treatment of this condition. The 'bold' variant of psychopathy is associated with fearlessness; situations that elicit fear in most people are experienced by bold psychopaths as exciting and thrilling. It was suggested that when boldness is combined with a callous and uncaring attitude toward others, it may be associated with a type of violence that is both impulsive (unpremeditated) and appetitively motivated (by a desire for excitement; see Figure 2.4) [27].

Epidemiology

In Chapter 5 we reviewed the epidemiology of ASPD. Several conclusions can be drawn from this. First, ASPD and PCL-R psychopathy are much more prevalent among criminal than among community samples. This is hardly surprising since, as indicated above, both constructs conflate personality variables with criminality. If they are to be meaningful psychological constructs, they need to be stripped of their association with criminal behaviour.

Second, ASPD is strongly associated with being young, male and socially disadvantaged. Men so diagnosed bear several disadvantages, including being poorly educated, having a low income and being single. They also suffer from multiple comorbidities, among which the most significant is alcohol and drug misuse. We suggest it is their drug and alcohol misuse that is largely responsible for these individuals falling into the net of the criminal justice system and particularly for their engaging in violent behaviour.

Third, few of these disadvantaged young men seek any treatment, and when they do it is largely because of co-occurring psychiatric disorders. In the language of Tyrer and colleagues [28] they are treatment rejecting rather than treatment seeking. We saw in the chapters dealing with treatment approaches that individuals with ASPD represent a significant challenge to anyone who seeks to intervene to alter their life's trajectory.

Finally, notwithstanding its greater prevalence in both male offenders and community residents, ASPD occurs in a substantial minority of the female population, with a higher prevalence (0.5–1%) in North American women than in European women <0.5%, and in a substantial proportion of female offenders [29]. Differences in the way that ASPD presents in men and women (see Table 1 in [29]) imply that criteria and thresholds for identifying ASPD might need to be adjusted to take account of these differences. Given the extent to which the profile of ASPD – its antecedents, criminological correlates and symptoms – is gender-specific, it is probably justifiable to talk about male and female *variants* of ASPD.

Treatment of ASPD

In Chapters 6 and 7 we reviewed approaches to treatment of individuals with a diagnosis of ASPD, first of all (Chapter 6) in community (non-specialist) settings and then (Chapter 7) in specialist settings where patients present with high needs and as high risk. In Chapter 6 we emphasised the importance of non-specific rather than specific factors in effecting a favourable outcome in psychotherapy. We recommended a stepped-care approach that comprises three consecutive phases: first, establishing therapeutic engagement; second, managing behavioural disturbance; and third, integration of self-states (Figure 6.1). We emphasised the need for the therapist to anticipate possible ruptures to the therapeutic process and to address these proactively. Production of a case formulation (discussed further below) at an early stage is considered essential.

In Chapter 7, we focused on the reduction of criminality and violence in those with 'severe ASPD' and psychopathy who may be detained in secure hospitals or incarcerated in prisons. The principles of the risk-needs-responsivity (RNR) and the Good Lives Model (GLM, discussed further below) were considered and contrasted. Finally, the management of those who are deemed beyond treatment was examined and its implications discussed. We outlined a set of general principles that should be followed. We emphasised that those with severe personality disorder, particularly where psychopathic features are salient, present a significant therapeutic challenge and that the objective of the intervention may need to focus more on risk reduction than on significant personality change. We also emphasised the need for a clear and explicit treatment strategy to be adopted and for the various professionals involved to commit to the strategy.

Legal and Ethical Issues

In Chapter 8 we explored the legal and ethical issues associated with the involuntary detention of offenders with antisocial personality disorder/psychopathy for treatment in either a secure hospital or prison. We charted the recent history and changing attitudes toward the compulsory detention of such individuals in the United Kingdom, and critically examined the notion of treatability and risk prediction, the two main determinants of such a process. We concluded with some recommendations on how such individuals should be managed in the future. We favour a complete uncoupling of health and criminal justice systems, and we examined some important consequences of this. We proposed that any remanded prisoner should not be assessed pre-sentence on the grounds that this would complicate the sentencing process and encourage the remanded individual to exaggerate their symptoms to avoid a prison disposal. Instead, we advocated that offenders be assessed after they have been sentenced and – provided such treatment is considered likely to make a difference – that they be offered treatment on a voluntary basis. Once the treatment has been completed, the individual would be returned to prison or – if at the end of their sentence – be discharged to the community.

Assessment of Antisocial Individuals: A Way Forward

It is clear that there is scope for improving the existing conceptualisation for PD and the methods used to assess it. It has been argued that serving a *clinical* goal of aiding practitioners in identifying, conceptualizing and treating conditions may be (increasingly) separate from a productive *research* classification [30]. We concur with this sentiment and propose that a *clinical*, in contrast to a research, assessment of PD needs to address the three aspects of self which we have considered earlier: self as social actor, self as motivated agent and self as autobiographical author. Assessment of antisocial personality should consider these three aspects of self. First, one needs a comprehensive assessment of traits to assess 'self as social actor'. This should include traits across all domains, not just traits associated with ASPD. Wygant and colleagues [31] usefully suggested that *moving away from predefined personality constellations to a descriptive approach based on individual trait profiles . . . may eventually prove more useful clinically and allow for better construct validity.*

No matter how these traits are measured, be it an instrument linked to DSM-5 Section 3 or to ICD-11, the results should be represented graphically so that the clinician is able to identify at a glance the overall pattern of traits. To the maximum extent possible, trait facets and sub-facets should be examined in order to reveal lower-order traits within the hierarchy that may be informative for generating a nuanced and personalized case formulation and treatment plan [12].

The second aspect of PD that needs to be assessed is 'self as motivated agent'. Here there is a need to develop an interview-based procedure that systematically probes the individual's values, goals and aspirations (this overlaps with GLM, outlined below). A useful adjunct to this interview would be measures of self-directedness obtained from Livesley's General Assessment of Personality Disorder (GAPD), a self-report instrument having two main scales, 'self pathology' and 'interpersonal problems'. GAPD scores have been found to differentiate PD from normal personality and other mental disorders and to distinguish between different levels of PD severity [32, 33]. It is as yet unclear to what extent GAPD might be able to distinguish PDs with a greater degree of antisociality from other PDs, but the prosocial scale within GAPD 'interpersonal problems' (would never sacrifice self to help someone else; avoids helping other people; does not see anything wrong with taking advantage of someone who is easily conned) might be useful in this regard.

Self-directedness in GAPD assesses (1) problems in setting and attaining rewarding personal goals and (2) feelings that there is a lack of meaning, purpose and direction (LMPD) to life. The LMPD scale, which appears to capture the construct of emptiness, discussed earlier in relation to boredom proneness, includes four items: (1) nothing that I do seems to have much purpose; (2) I drift through life without a clear sense of direction; (3) my life seems to have little meaning; and (4) most of the time I feel that what I do is meaningful and valuable (reverse scored). A recent study [34] found that LMPD was significantly higher in PD patients than in patients lacking a PD diagnosis and healthy controls; moreover, LMPD score was significantly associated with a lack of affiliative relationships measured by GAPD. An important clinical implication of this study was that the exploration of feelings of meaninglessness and emptiness should be part of the assessment of PD. Again, it is not clear from this study whether patients with ASPD scored especially high on LMPD, since ASPD was not well represented in the sample and, as we saw in Chapter 7, people with ASPD are very focused on what they want, to their own and others' disadvantage. The association of LMPD with a lack of affiliative relationships implies that to have a sense of direction and meaning in one's life one must be locked into a network of social relationships.

The third aspect of antisocial personality that needs to be assessed is narrative identity. Important life-story constructs that might be assessed have been outlined by McAdams and McLean [35]. The degree of agency manifested in stories – the degree to which they privilege accomplishment and the ability to control one's fate – appears to be an especially important construct with regard to mental health. We suggest that an interview assessing values, goals and aspirations might be combined with an interview-based assessment of narrative identity. This might loosely be based on the procedure used by See and colleagues to examine narrative identity in schizotypal youth [36]. These authors coded turning-point narratives for three dimensions: agency, self-event connections and redemption – as well as schizotypal PD (STPD) symptoms. Since we are primarily interested in antisocial personality, this interview protocol would need to be adapted, for example, by substituting 'ASPD-like symptoms' for 'STPD-like symptoms', and perhaps using an alternative to the turning-point scenario.

The fourth and final element in the assessment would aim to locate the individual on the prosocial-antisocial continuum. This would be on a scale of 0 to 10, ranging from prosocial (0) to severely antisocial (10). This assessment would be based both on the trait assessment and on the assessment of motivated agent and personal narrative aspects of self. A high (antisocial) score would apply to someone who showed:

1. Widespread personality pathology across several trait domains (e.g., in ICD-11, disinhibition, negative affectivity and dissociality). Particular attention should be paid to the presence of *paranoid traits* as a marker for violence risk.
2. Evidence of severely disturbed behaviour starting in early childhood and continuing into adolescence, particularly if accompanied by misuse of alcohol and drugs.
3. A dysfunctional motivational agenda showing either deviant or unrealistic goals, values and aspirations.
4. A disturbed narrative identity, for example, one that lacks a clear sense of agency (the ability to effect change in their lives and influence others in their environment) and sense of communion (intimacy, caring and belongingness).

Clearly, much work needs to be done in developing a suitable interview protocol that meets these objectives.

From Assessment to Case Formulation

As we outlined in Chapters 6 and 7, a case formulation needs to be developed that is grounded in the above assessments in order to create an understanding of the individual as they are now. The case formulation addresses the whole person, seeking to articulate the central mechanisms that cause and maintain their main problems and explain how the problems are related [37]. Developmental processes are described together with the functions that the individual's problem behaviours have for the individual. In the case of an individual showing violent behaviour, it is important that the case formulation identifies the *type* of violence that is shown and the *functions* it serves. We saw in Chapter 3 that emotion goals can vary according to the motivation underlying the individual's violence: a desire for excitement and thrills (when feeling bored), a desire for safety (when feeling interpersonally threatened), a desire for vengeance (when feeling aggrieved and resentful) or a desire for self-gratification (when feeling greedy and concupiscent). We emphasise that these goals are not inherently antisocial; it is *the violent means used to attain them*, not the goals themselves, that are antisocial. Attainment of these emotion goals may equally be sought in prosocial ways. Alternative means of goal attainment can subsequently be explored with the client, for example, how they might learn to cope in a prosocial way with feelings of boredom or resentment. We emphasise also the importance of considering how violence is cognitively framed through a process of moral disengagement, said by Caprara and colleagues to be 'the gatekeeper that makes harmful behavior accessible without incurring self-blame and painful emotions' [25, p. 80].

The case formulation also seeks to identify what treatments are likely to be effective, ineffective or even – as we discussed in Chapters 6 and 7 – harmful. Consistent with the Good Lives Model (GLM) discussed below, it is important that positive aspects are included in a strength-based case formulation, covering areas such as work, relationships, accommodation, health and leisure activities. As discussed by Sturmey and colleagues [37], an adequate case formulation should, first, tell a coherent, ordered and meaningful story; second, it should be consistent with an empirically supported theory; third, it should be based on an adequate amount of good-quality, relevant information about the past and the present that is tied together to show relationships; and last, it should go beyond simple description to make detailed and testable predictions about which strategies will be most effective in treating and managing harmful behaviour.

Approaches to Rehabilitation and Treatment

The approach to rehabilitation of offenders that sits most comfortably with the type of assessment we have proposed above is the Good Lives Model (GLM) developed by Ward and colleagues [38]. GLM was previously discussed briefly in connection with treatment of ASPD in Chapter 6, but it is important to note here that GLM is neither a comprehensive theory of offending behaviour nor a treatment model. Although the evidence supporting GLM is very preliminary, its approach to rehabilitation is grounded in the important idea that engaging offenders and motivating them to change is conditional on offering them the possibility of a better life. Its premise is that all meaningful human actions represent attempts to secure *primary human goods* (PHGs), overarching life pursuits or ultimate concerns that are expressed in the many and varied goals that we set for ourselves (we might refer to PHGs as 'meta-goals'). According to GLM there are 10 PHGs: *knowledge, excellence in play, excellence in work, excellence in agency, inner peace, relatedness, community, spirituality, pleasure, creativity*. Most importantly, GLM argues that people offend in the pursuit of PHGs, *but do so in harmful ways due to their individual set of internal and external deficits and obstacles*. Its approach to rehabilitation is essentially to shift the individual along the antisocial-prosocial continuum in a prosocial direction by increasing their internal capacity and skills and increasing their external resources and social support. The aim of rehabilitation is to identify what problems exist so that lifestyles and life plans can be altered to suit each offender's preferences, capabilities, skills, temperament and opportunities. As stated by Purvis and Ward, 'The aim of rehabilitation, therefore, is to build and add to individuals' social and psychological resources. In this way, we increase and improve the person's capacity, choice, opportunity, well-being and outcomes. This building up of the person then allows the individual to access goods in pro-social ways that are also intrinsically beneficial and meaningful' [38].

We can illustrate the core principles of GLM with reference to patient Y, whom we encountered in Chapter 7. Recall that Y was a shy and introverted young man who had difficulties in establishing close and intimate relationships with members of the opposite sex, despite wanting to do so. We can assume that the meta-goal of 'relatedness' was high in his hierarchy of PHGs, as was his meta-goal of 'excellence in agency' (his need for autonomy, self-directedness, personal power, control and mastery). There were a number of obstacles, both internal and external, to his achieving satisfaction of his need to relate to members of the opposite sex. Internal impediments included his lack of interpersonal skills, his distrust of others, and an inability to control his emotional impulses, together with a lack of a sense of personal agency. At the time of his offence, and despite his evident talents, he lacked the type of work that might have given him a sense of achievement and fulfilment. Psychological impediments might have included a lack of self-belief and motivation to achieve (and perhaps a lack of insight into his own behaviour). His problem was that he sought the good of relatedness by adopting inappropriate means, for example, by forming a romantic attachment to his psychologist. External impediments included a lack of opportunity, through employment or education, to realise his potential as a musician, and his social isolation. Y's offence – the poisoning of his work colleagues – arose in the context of emotional turmoil. It was an inappropriate and misguided attempt to obtain emotional equilibrium (i.e., inner peace) by terminating the unpleasant emotional states arising from his colleagues' derogatory and sexually explicit remarks about the female colleague with whom he had developed a relationship.

As we saw in Chapter 6, the long-term outcome in Y's case was positive – he managed to overcome the internal and external obstacles to achieving success both in work and in his interpersonal relationships. Through a mixture of psychotherapy and his own efforts, he achieved the good of 'excellence in work' by gaining skills in musicianship and instrument making. He found meaning and purpose in life and achieved an inner peace. In short, he moved toward the prosocial end of the antisocial-prosocial continuum by increasing his internal capacity and skills and increasing his external resources and social support.

Y exemplifies successful *desistance* from criminal behaviour. Maruna identified that 'to desist from crime, ex-offenders need to develop a coherent, pro-social identity for themselves' [**39**, p. 7]. This derives from his finding that individuals who were able to desist from crime had high levels of self-efficacy, meaning that they saw themselves in control of their futures and had a clear sense of purpose and meaning in their lives. They also found a way to 'make sense' out of their past lives and even find some redeeming value in lives that had often been spent in and out of prisons and jails. In a similar vein, Ward has emphasised the significant role played by *agency* in desistance, reflecting the individual's unique viewpoint [**40**]. According to Ward's *Predictive Agency Model of Protective Factors* (PAMP), these are best understood as internal and external capacities that enable individuals to realize valued outcomes in prosocial ways. Ward argues that practitioners should use techniques and strategies that are likely to provide individuals with the capacities and resources to engage in productive agency. Importantly, and in keeping with the treatment approach we have advocated in Chapters 6 and 7, this approach places importance on the *process* or *relationship* aspects of intervention, emphasising in particular the need to develop strong relationships with clients.

In terms of treatment, a critical question is whether a GLM-informed treatment programme would show improved outcomes, in particular, lower rates of recidivism, when compared with programmes that simply focus on risk reduction (i.e., are informed only by risk-needs-responsivity [RNR] principles). Such studies are virtually nonexistent, but exceptionally one study did make a relevant comparison between two treatments in incarcerated sex offenders [**41**]. A control group comprised untreated sex offenders. One intervention was a standard sex offender treatment programme that focused on risk reduction. The other was a strengths-based approach that emphasised the benefits of building a better life; it 'was offered as a way to not only reduce the likelihood of reoffending but also provide the strengths needed to have a better, more fulfilling future' [**41**, p. 6]. Importantly, toward the end of the strengths-based treatment participants were assisted in developing future plans aimed at further enhancing their strengths in the areas of education and work skills. The GLM-informed treatment group showed significantly lower rates of sexual and violent recidivism compared with the standard sex offender treatment programme group, as well as lower drop-out rates. While not a randomized control trial, this study was carefully conducted and controlled for risk through stratified group comparisons (low vs medium vs high risk).

Post-Script

Throughout this book, we have attempted to chart a middle path, avoiding both the Scylla of diagnostic nihilism and the Charybdis of being straitjacketed within the confines of a narrow medical model that assumes symptom (or trait) profiles are meaningful indicators of the nature of some underlying disorder [42]. We acknowledge that it may be useful and necessary to consider extremes of personality as falling within the purview of psychiatry. On the other hand, we acknowledge, with Fischer [43], that there is a regrettable separation of the clinical field of PD from other disciplines, psychology in particular, that may provide important new insights into clinical practice and training. We hope that the reader will be convinced by the authors' argument that emotion and motivation lie at the heart of antisocial personality and that this extends beyond the confines of constructs – antisocial personality *disorder* and psychopathy – with which it has traditionally been associated. We have emphasized in particular the importance of considering the motivational and emotional underpinnings of antisocial personality, underscoring the importance of feelings such as distrust and paranoia, boredom, greed, vengeance and insecurity as mainsprings of antisocial behaviour.

References

1. D. Westen, J. Shedler, B. Bradley, J. A. DeFife. An empirically derived taxonomy for personality disorders: Bridging science and practice in conceptualising personality. *American Journal of Psychiatry* 2012; **169**: 273–284.

2. L. Smith Benjamin. *Interpersonal Diagnosis and Treatment of Personality Disorders*. New York: Guilford Press, 1996.

3. C. M. Strickland, C. J Hopwood, M. A. Bornavolova, E. C. Rojas. Categorical and dimensional conceptions of personality pathology in DSM-5: Toward a model-based synthesis. *Journal of Personality Disorders* 2019; **33**: 185–213.

4. L. J. Cronbach, P. E. Meehl. Construct validity in psychological tests. *Psychological Bulletin* 1955; **52**: 281–302.

5. S. O. Lilienfeld, A. L. Watts, B. Murphy, T. H. Costello, S. M. Bowes, S. F. Smith, R. D. Latzman, N. Haslam, K. Tabb. Personality disorders as emergent interpersonal syndromes: Psychopathic personality as a case example. *Journal of Personality Disorders* 2019; **33**: 577–622.

6. J. W. Coid, M. Yang, S. Ullrich, T. Zhang, S. Sizmur, D. Farrington, R. Rogers. Most items in structured risk assessment instruments do not predict violence. *Journal of Forensic Psychiatry and Psychology* 2011; **22**: 3–21.

7. H. Hawkins-Elder, T. Ward. Describing disorder: The importance and advancement of compositional explanations in psychopathology. *Theory & Psychology* 2021; in press.

8. A. C. Helle, K. J. Sher, T. J. Trull. Individual symptoms or categorical diagnoses? An epidemiological examination of the association between alcohol use, personality disorders, and psychological symptoms. *Personality Disorders: Theory, Research, and Treatment*. Advance online publication. https://doi.org/10.1037/per0000459.

9. T. Rosenström, F. A. Torvik, E. Ystrom, N. O. Czajkowski, N. A. Gillespie, S. H. Aggen, R. F. Krueger, K. S Kendler, T. Reichborn-Kjennerud. Prediction of alcohol use disorder using personality disorder traits: A twin study. *Addiction* 2018; **113**: 15–24.

10. C. E. Vize, K. L. Collison, D. R. Lynam. The importance of antagonism: Explaining similarities and differences in psychopathy and narcissism's relations with aggression and externalizing outcomes. *Journal of Personality Disorders* 2020; **34**: 1–13.

11. F. Gutiérrez, E. Vicente, A. Aluja, J. M. Peri, A. Gutiérrez-Zotes, E. Baillés, S. E. Villamon, M. A. R. Rodríguez, A. M. de Alba, G. Vall, D. Gallardo-Pujol. Dimensional Assessment of Personality Pathology – Basic Questionnaire. *Personality and Mental Health* 2021; 1–13.

12. A. G. C. Wright, W. C. Woods. Personalized models of psychopathology. *Annual Review of Clinical Psychology* 2020; **16**: 49–74.

13. S. R. Masland, T. V. Shah, L. W. Choi-Kain. Boredom in borderline personality disorder: A lost criterion reconsidered. *Psychopathology* 2020; **53**: 239–253.

14. J. Mugon, J. Boylan, J. Danckert. Boredom proneness and self-control as unique risk factors in achievement settings. *International Journal of Environmental Research and Public Health* 2020; **17**: 9116.

15. K. Y. Y. Tam, W. A. P. van Tilburg, C. S. Chan. What is boredom proneness? A comparison of three characterizations. *Journal of Personality* 2021; doi: 10.1111/jopy.12618.

16. A. Konjusha, C. J. Hopwood, A. L. Price, O. Masuhr, J. Zimmermann. Investigating the transdiagnostic value of subjective emptiness. *Journal of Personality Disorders*, https://doi.org/10.1521/pedi_2021_35_510.

17. J. Eastwood, V. Bambrah. Self-focused but lacking in self-knowledge. The relation between boredom and self-perception. Paper presented at the online 4th International Boredom Conference, 24–26 June 2021.

18. J. E. Muñoz-Negro, C. Prudent, B. Gutiérrez, J. Cervilla. Paranoia and risk of personality disorder in the general population. *Personality and Mental Health* 2019; **13**: 107–116. doi: 10.1002/pmh.1511.

18. M. McMurran, G. Christopher. Dysfunctional beliefs and antisocial personality disorder. *The Journal of Forensic Psychiatry & Psychology* 2008; **19**: 533–542.

19. N. Raihani, D. Martinez-Gatell, V. Bell, L. Foulkes. Social reward, punishment, and prosociality in paranoia. *Journal of Abnormal Psychology* 2021; 130: 177–185. http://dx.doi.org/10.1037/abn0000647.

20. A. Trotta , J. Kang, D. Stahl, J. Yiend. Interpretation bias in paranoia: A systematic review and meta-analysis. *Clinical Psychological Science* 2021; **9**: 3–23.

21. C. L. M. Lam, E. Mouchlianitis, T. M. C. Lee, J. Yiend. Anxiety mediates the relationship between interpretation bias and paranoia in patients with persistent persecutory beliefs. *Anxiety, Stress & Coping. An International Journal* 2021; **34**: 96–106. doi: 10.1080/10615806.2020.1802435.

22. L. H. Grobbink, J. J. L. Derksen, H. J. C. van Marle. Revenge: An analysis of its psychological underpinnings. *International Journal of Offender Therapy and Comparative Criminology* 2014; **59**: 892–907.

23. W. C. Myers, E. Lee, R. Montplaisir, E. Lazarou, M. Safarik, H. C. Chan, E. Beauregard. Revenge filicide: An international perspective through 62 cases. *Behavioral Sciences and the Law* 2021; **39**: 205–215.

24. E. A. Selby, T. E. Joiner. Cascades of emotion: The emergence of borderline personality disorder from emotion and behavioural dysregulation. *Review of General Psychology* 2009; **13**: 219–229.

25. G. V. Caprara, M. S. Tisak, G. Alessandri, R. G. Fontaine, R. Fida, M. Paciello. The contribution of moral disengagement in mediating individual tendencies toward aggression and violence. *Developmental Psychology* 2014; **50**: 71–85.

26. C. Martinelli, K. Cavanagh, R. E. J. Dudley. The impact of rumination on state paranoid ideation in a nonclinical sample. *Behavior Therapy* 2013; **44**: 385–394.

27. R. C. Howard. Psychopathy, impulsiveness and violence: How are they linked? *Journal of Behavior* 2017; **2**: 1004.

28. P. Tyrer, S. Mitchard, C. Methuen, M. Ranger. Treatment rejecting and

treatment seeking personality disorders: Type R and type S. *Journal of Personality Disorders* 2003; **17**: 263–268.

29. B. Bishop, B. Völlm, N. Khalifa. Women with antisocial personality disorder. In: D. W. Black, N. Kolla, eds., *Textbook of Antisocial Personality Disorder*. Washington, DC: American Psychiatric Press, 2021.

30. R. K. Blashfield, J. W. Keeley, E. H. Flanagan, S. R. Miles. The cycle of classification: DSM-I through DSM-5. *Annual Review of Clinical Psychology* 2014; **10**: 25–51.

31. D. B. Wygant, M. Sellbom, C. E. Sleep, T. D. Wall, K. C. Applegate, R. F. Krueger, C. J. Patrick. Examining the DSM-5 alternative personality disorder model operationalization of antisocial personality disorder and psychopathy in a male correctional sample. *Personality Disorders: Theory, Research, and Treatment* 2016; **7**: 229–239. https://doi .org/10.1037/per0000179.

32. A. G. Hentschel, W. J. Livesley. Differentiating normal and disordered personality using the General Assessment of Personality Disorder (GAPD). *Personality and Mental Health* 2013; **7**: 133–142.

33. H. Berghuis, J. H. Kamphuis, R. Verheul, R. Larstone, W. J. Livesley. The General Assessment of Personality Disorder (GAPD) as an instrument for assessing the core features of personality disorders. *Clinical Psychology and Psychotherapy* 2012; **20**: 544–557.

34. A. Steen, H. Berghuis, A. W. Braam. Lack of meaning, purpose and direction in life in personality disorder: A comparative quantitative approach using Livesley's General Assessment of Personality Disorder. *Personality and Mental Health* 2019. doi 10.1002/pmh.1446.

35. D. P. McAdams, K. C. McLean. Narrative identity. *Current Directions in Psychological Science* 2013; **22**: 233.

36. A. Y. See, T. A. Klimstra, R. L. Shiner, J. J. A. Denissen. Linking narrative identity with schizotypal personality disorder features in adolescents. *Personality Disorders: Theory, Research, and Treatment*. Advance online publication. https://doi.org/10.1037/per0000414.

37. P. Sturmey, M. McMurran, M. Daffern. Case formulation and treatment planning. In: D. L. L. Polaschek, A. Day, C. R. Hollin, eds., *The Wiley International Handbook of Correctional Psychology*. Chichester: John Wiley & Sons, 2019; 476–487.

38. M. Purvis, T. Ward. An overview of the Good Lives Model: Theory and evidence. In: P. Ugwudike, H. Graham, F. McNeill, P. Raynor, F. S. Taxman, C. Trotter, eds., *The Routledge Companion to Rehabilitative Work in Criminal Justice*. New York: Routledge, 2020.

39. S. Maruna. *Making Good: How Ex-Convicts Reform and Rebuild Their Lives*. Washington, DC: American Psychological Association Books, 2001.

40. T. Ward. Prediction and agency: The role of protective factors in correctional rehabilitation and desistance. *Aggression and Violent Behavior* 2017; **32**: 19–28.

41. M. E. Olver , L. E. Marshall, W. L. Marshall, T. P. Nicholaichuk. A long-term outcome assessment of the effects on subsequent reoffense rates of a prison-based CBT/RNR sex offender treatment program with strength-based elements. *Sexual Abuse* 2020; **32**: 1–27.

42. C. E. Wilshire, T. Ward, S. Clack. Symptom descriptions in psychopathology: How well are they working for us? *Clinical Psychological Science*. 2020; **9**: 323–339.

43. R. Fischer. *Personality, Values, Culture: An Evolutionary Perspective*. Cambridge: Cambridge University Press, 2017.

Index

Printed in the United States
by Baker & Taylor Publisher Services